CW00971671

current
nursing
practice

Neuromedical and
Neurosurgical Nursing

Current Nursing Practice titles
(in preparation)

Neuromedical and Neurosurgical Nursing

Gillian Purchese, SRN
(Diploma in Neurological and Neurosurgical Nursing)
Formerly Sister-in-Charge
The Neurological and Neurosurgical Unit
The Middlesex Hospital, London

Douglas Allan, RGN, RMN
Charge Nurse, Intensive Therapy Unit
Institute of Neurological Sciences
Southern General Hospital, Glasgow

Second edition

Baillière Tindall London Philadelphia Toronto
Mexico City Rio de Janeiro Sydney Tokyo Hong Kong

Baillière Tindall   1 St Anne's Road
Eastbourne, East Sussex BN21 3UN, England

West Washington Square
Philadelphia, PA 19105, U.S.A.

1 Goldthorne Avenue
Toronto, Ontario M8Z 5T9, Canada

Apartado 26370—Cedro 512
Mexico 4, D.F., Mexico

Rua Evaristo da Veiga, 55—20° andar
Rio de Janeiro — RJ, Brazil

ABP Australia Ltd, 44 Waterloo Road
North Ryde, NSW 2064, Australia

Ichibancho Central Building, 22–1 Ichibancho
Chiyoda-ku, Tokyo 102, Japan

10/FL, Inter-Continental Plaza, 94 Granville Road
Tsim Sha Tsui East, Kowloon, Hong Kong

First published as Nurses' Aids Series Special Interest Text 1977
Second edition 1984

Typeset by Inforum Ltd, Portsmouth
Printed in Great Britain by
Richard Clay (The Chaucer Press) Ltd
Bungay, Suffolk

British Library Cataloguing in Publication Data

Purchese, Gillian
  Neuromedical and neurosurgical nursing.—2nd ed.
  —(Current nursing practice)
  1. Neurological nursing
  I. Title   II. Allan, Douglas   III. Series
  616.8'024613   RC350.5

  ISBN 0–7020–1030–8

Contents

Preface

I am delighted and privileged to have been allowed the opportunity to revise Miss Purchese's original edition of *Neuromedical and Neurosurgical Nursing*.

Nursing is rapidly emerging as a profession distinct from medicine, and it follows that nurses are the only people qualified to define and commit to paper their body of knowledge. It was with this concept in mind that this text was revised. Changes made include an expansion of the sections on related nursing skills and on the extended role of the nurse; comprehensive reading lists have been added at the end of each chapter to satisfy the appetite of the reader who wishes to explore further into a particular aspect of neurological nursing; and updated methods of treating patients are also included, some of which remain in the early stages of research.

Douglas Allan

Acknowledgements

I would like to express my deepest gratitude to Mr Y. Kohi, Senior Neurosurgical Registrar, and Dr I. Bone, Consultant Neurologist, both of the Institute of Neurological Sciences, Glasgow, who advised on the neurosurgical and neuromedical aspects respectively; and to all my nursing colleagues at the institute, who are too numerous to mention by name, who advised, criticised and encouraged my endeavours, in particular the staff of the intensive therapy unit (who covered up for me during my visits to the library) and Mr J. Smith, previously Nursing Officer, Theatres.

I would like to acknowledge the permission given by the Editor of *Nursing Times* for the reproduction of Figs. 2.2 and 2.4.

I am indebted to the librarians of the Central Library for Professional Staff at the Southern General Hospital, and the South-East and South-West Districts Colleges of Nursing libraries, Greater Glasgow Health Board.

Mention should be made of the contributions made by Miss E. Grainger (dietetics), Mrs S. Wade (social work) and Mr D. McNiven and staff (physiotherapy). I am indebted to Mrs G. Galbraith and my wife Morag who typed the script, and to Miss R. Long and staff at Baillière Tindall.

Last, but not least, I would like to thank my wife and son for patiently tolerating my long absences from home, my bad moods and the pieces of paper that were left scattered over the house; they persevered with this project long after I had given up.

Douglas Allan

1 Neurological nursing

Neurological nursing involves caring for those patients suffering from disorders of the nervous system, which can arise as a result of trauma, congenital malformations, blood vessel disorders, malignant and benign tumours, infections and degenerative disorders. Some patients will be admitted to hospital, investigated and offered surgery or drug therapy in order to alleviate their complaints, and will eventually be discharged home with or without a varying degree of disability. Others may be offered only palliative treatment and arrangements made for the appropriate terminal nursing care. A third group of patients will be admitted or re-admitted during the course of a chronic degenerative neurological disorder, requiring meticulous nursing intervention and suitable community support on discharge.

The nervous system is perhaps the most complex and difficult to understand, and no other system affects the functioning of other parts of the body as much as it does. The nurse often needs to deal with the physical manifestations of a disorder of the nervous system as well as the neurological dysfunction itself, which explains the high ratio of dependent patients found within neurological centres. In most cases the overriding clinical consideration is the patient's level of consciousness, which can range from full alertness and orientation with no obvious major deficits, to being deeply unconscious and fully dependent on others to provide basic physical needs. Between these two extremes is a full range of patients who may display physical disabilities with no clouding of consciousness or mental states, and, conversely, those who display psychiatric symptoms and no obvious physical handicap.

Considerable challenges are created by this very wide spectrum of patients, and the nurse can derive immense personal satisfaction from helping a very ill, unconscious patient, requiring an infinite degree of nursing care, to get better and return home to rejoin his family. If the patient is to achieve his maximum potential following an accident or illness, meticulous attention to the details of basic nursing procedures is absolutely essential, and this can be achieved only by good bedside nursing. The way in which an unconscious patient's limbs are positioned will ultimately determine how well that patient may walk once recovery is complete.

All the staff caring for the patient rely on the nurse's keen perception and continuous observations; in particular, doctors greatly value a skilled nursing team which maintains advised treatments and reports changes in the patient's condition. The broad spectrum of symptomatology can provide an enormous challenge when it comes to planning nursing care, and the development and progress of the Nursing Process has a huge potential within the realm of neuromedical and neurosurgical nursing.

The Nursing Process

The Nursing Process was devised in order to provide the optimum nursing care, developed in a rational and effective manner. There are four stages to the Process: the first involves assessing the patient to determine what nursing care, if any, he may require. The assessment will consist of collecting data from the patient, which will include obtaining a nursing history. A pre-prepared questionnaire is probably the easiest way for the nurse to elicit the information needed.

Various models have been developed, and whichever one is used will depend on local policy. Many are centered on the Activities of Daily Living (ADL): one such example is the Roper model, based on 12 modes of behaviour, i.e. the ability to maintain a safe environment, communication skills, breathing, eating and drinking, elimination, personal cleansing, control of body temperature, mobility, work and play, expressing sexuality, sleep routine, and attitude to death.

The second stage involves analysing the data and then deciding how to nurse the patient. At this point, a written nursing care plan is created and its contents made known to all members of the team caring for the patient. Implementation of the nursing care comprises the third stage in the process, and evaluation of that nursing care and its effects constitutes the fourth stage. It should be borne in mind that the assessment is a continuous process, and that changes will need to be made in the light of new developments or ineffectual nursing care.

Advances in diagnosis and treatment have been greater in the field of nervous disorders than in almost any other medical specialty. The continued development and availability of computerised axial tomography (CT scan) enhances patient care by offering a hazard-free, non-invasive technique for obtaining clear pictures of the intracranial contents and those of other body cavities. Other, newer developments within the diagnostic field include the emergence of the positron emission scanner and the nuclear magnetic resonance scanner.

Better methods and improved interpretation of data from intracranial pressure monitoring allow more rapid and effective intervention in head-injured patients. The advent of the operating microscope and a greater understanding of cerebral blood flow have created a new avenue of treatment for patients suffering from previously inoperable neurovascular disorders. Improved methods of pain relief have allowed terminally ill patients to die painlessly and drug free, and have created a small subgroup of nurses specialising in the administration of these new techniques.

The development of neurological intensive care areas, with their sophisticated monitoring systems and ventilatory equipment, has provided the nurse with new challenges for the future, not least of which concern the ethical considerations. A modern by-product of these new techniques which we have now to come to terms with is cerebral death. Patients who would previously have not survived their injuries are now resuscitated more effectively in the early hours following their accident, but unfortunately some survive merely to die 48–72 hours later. The methodology used to determine cerebral death is discussed in the Appendix.

FURTHER READING

KRATZ, C. (ed.) (1979) *The Nursing Process*. London: Baillière Tindall.
LONG, R. (1981) *Systematic Nursing Care*. London: Faber and Faber.
ROPER, N., LOGAN, W.W. & TIERNEY, A.J. (1980) *The Elements of Nursing*. Edinburgh: Churchill Livingstone.
ROPER, N., LOGAN, W.W. & TIERNEY, A.J. (1981) *Learning to Use the Process of Nursing*. Edinburgh: Churchill Livingstone.
ROPER, N., LOGAN, W.W. & TIERNEY, A.J. (1983) *Using a Model for Nursing*. Edinburgh: Churchill Livingstone.
WEST, A. (1980) Patient into person (nursing process). *Nursing Mirror, 150*:8, 32.
WILLE, R.L. (1979) Neurosurgical nursing: past, present and future. *Heart and Lung, 8*:5, 819.

2 Admission and assessment

For most people, admission to hospital, either electively or as an emergency, is a traumatic experience. The associated stress can be reduced by the admitting nurse's attitude and a relaxation of rigid hospital rules that appear to have been designed to depersonalise the individual. The welcome of the patient is a crucial part of his hospitalisation, as his initial impression will probably be his most vivid. The nurse who admits the patient must combine friendliness and a helpful attitude with keen observation and an accurate recording of facts. The relatives will also feel reassured if the nurse is attentive and sympathetic.

The priorities which determine the usual admission procedure are dictated by the nature of the patient's illness. Patients for elective admission have had time to consider its implications, and will have made special arrangements in respect of their personal life and work commitments. They will appear for admission at a convenient pre-arranged time and date, and the ward sister will usually receive advance notice in order to allow her to make arrangements within the ward so that the admission proceeds smoothly.

However, the emergency admission procedure is quite different. Very little warning will be given, and often the information is scanty, therefore those departments, i.e. ITU and high dependency units, which regularly receive patients under these circumstances will be in a state of readiness on their admission days. A bed isolated from perceptive patients will be required with the necessary equipment assembled ready for use. This equipment will include oxygen and suction, airways, Ambu resuscitator bag, equipment for intubation and the setting up of intravenous fluids, a nasogastric tube, and a basic monitoring system to include cardiac and respiratory functions. There should also be access to ventilatory and emergency resuscitation equipment.

An important aspect of admission is gathering data through the completion of a pre-prepared nursing history in order that an individual care plan can be drawn up for each patient. The structure of the questionnaire can be based on the activities of daily living (ADL) and should cover:

maintaining a safe environment
communication
breathing
eating and drinking
elimination
personal hygiene and dressing
controlling body temperature
mobilisation
work and social habits
expressing sexuality
sleeping
dying

Information will also be sought in respect of the next of kin and other significant relatives and friends, the patient's own knowledge and perception of his illness and admission to hospital.

If an unconscious patient is received with, for example, a severe head injury, then the process requires some modification as communication with the patient will be impossible. Information can be gleaned from medical and nursing notes taken on admission to the A and E department, talking with the nurse or doctor who accompanied the patient, interviewing relatives (if present), and performing a physical assessment of the patient. The use of a pre-prepared questionnaire (Fig. 2.1) will reduce the time taken to perform the assessment, as also will the adoption of a standardised coma scale such as the Glasgow Coma Scale.

The Glasgow Coma Scale

The Glasgow Coma Scale (Fig. 2.2) was devised to provide a standard method of measuring the level of consciousness in a patient. It eliminates the problems caused by the use of ambiguous terms such as semicomatose and stupor. The scale is based on assessing three modes of behaviour — eye opening, verbal response, and motor response — and is designed for use by all grades of personnel. Each mode of behaviour is assessed independently and charted on an easy-to-follow form. Any deterioration will be quickly demonstrated as a downward trend.

Name _____ Diagnosis _____

Dentures   YES/NO   Removed   YES/NO   Family present   YES/NO
Seen by Doctor   YES/NO

Neuro. Glasgow Coma Scale: Eyes opening_____
                           Best verbal response _____
                           Best motor response _____

Pupils: Right _____ mm. NRTL   Left _____ mm. NRTL

Limb movements: *Left Right*   *Left Right*
             Legs: Normal Power   Arms: Normal Power
                   Mild Weakness   Mild Weakness
                   Severe Weakness   Severe Weakness
                   Extension   Spastic Weakness
                   No Response   Spastic Flexion
                                           Extension
                                           No Response

Pulmonary: Spon. Resp. Rate _____ Airway _____ Intubated _____
Size of tube _____

O₂ via _____ FiO₂ _____ Ambu bag present YES/NO
Ventilator: TV _____ R _____ FiO₂ _____
Suctioned _____ Character _____
Gastro-
   intestinal: Naso-gastric Tube YES/NO   Character of Drainage __
Genito-Urinary: Urinary Catheter   YES/NO   Urine _____
IV Fluids: Solution
                              Additives   Amt. Remaining

              a) _____
              b) _____
              c) _____
CVP _____
Other Invasive Lines: e.g. Arterial Lines _____
Other Injuries (Briefly summarise, to include Abrasions, Lacerations,
   Soft Tissue injuries and Fractures)

Skull: _____
Facial: _____
Chest: _____
Abdomen: _____
Orthopaedic: _____

Fig. 2.1. *Intensive therapy unit patient profile form.*

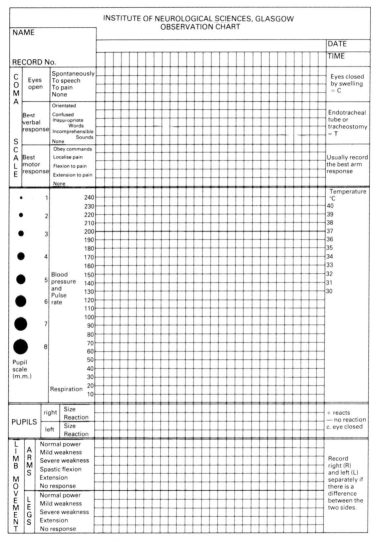

Fig. 2.2. *Glasgow Coma Scale.*

Eye opening

> Spontaneously
> To speech
> To pain
> None

The degree of stimulation required to make the patient open his eyes is tested. As the nurse approaches the patient, she should observe whether his eyes are open or closed. If the patient's eyes are closed, then calling the patient by name may elicit an eye-opening response, in which case the patient is said to be eye opening to speech. If, however, the patient still does not open his eyes, a painful stimuli will have to be applied. The easiest way to do this is by exerting pressure on the proximal side of the nailbed (Fig. 2.3). Rubbing the sternum is not recommended. If the patient now opens his eyes, he is considered to be eye opening to pain, but should this stimulation fail, the patient is recorded as having no eye opening. One or two points need to be observed before the score can be applied. If the patient cannot open his eyes due to peri-orbital swelling, this is noted on the record as (C=closed) and not as no eye opening. On the other hand, an unconscious patient with flaccid eye

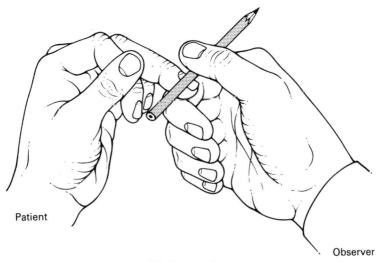

Fig. 2.3. *Finger-nail pressure.*

muscles may lie with his eyes open all the time once the lids have been retracted; this is recorded as no eye opening, as it is not a true arousal response.

Verbal response

  Orientated
  Confused conversation
  Inappropriate words
  Incomprehensible sounds
  No verbal response

The patient is questioned to determine that he is orientated to time, place and person. He should not be expected to answer absolutely correctly every time, and allowances are made for this. However, if a patient gives the completely wrong answers but is able to converse, this is recorded as confusion. At the next level down, the patient will speak only one or two words, usually obscenities, and this is termed inappropriate words. If only grunts or moans are obtained in response to a painful stimulus, this is described as incomprehensible sounds. A complete lack of verbal response is recorded as such. Factors which may alter the outcome of results in this section of the scale include:

  a. the patient's inability to understand the assessor's commands, either because of a hearing deficit or an inability to comprehend the native language;
  b. the presence of an endotracheal or tracheostomy tube will prevent phonation, and this is recorded in the chart as T;
  c. the existence of a speech difficulty, e.g. aphasia.

Motor response

  Obeys commands
  Localisation
  Flexion
  Extension
  No response

To assess if a patient will obey commands, he is requested to perform a simple task, such as sticking his tongue out or lifting his hands up, and then his response is gauged. If the patient will not do this, painful stimulus is applied to the supra-orbital ridge, and the response observed. If the patient locates to the focus of irritation and attempts to remove it, or if he raises his hands up as far as his chin or higher, he is considered to be localising. If the patient does not localise, then finger-nail stimulation is performed. Bending of the elbow and withdrawal of the hand is considered a flexion response; and, if the elbow straightens, this is termed an extension response. The wrists may also internally rotate, and indeed some patients may retain this posture with minimal or no stimulation. It is the *best* arm response that is recorded, even when the responses from the two sides are different. The leg responses are limited and, when present, may be due to a spinal reflex. The poorest level of this part of the scale is no response to painful stimulus.

Other factors may need to be taken into consideration when evaluating the unconscious patient, and these can be charted with the coma scale, on the one form. These other parameters will detect local abnormalities as opposed to overall brain dysfunction. They include:

a.   vital signs
b.   observation of pupil size and reaction (Fig. 2.4), and limb movements.

a.   Vital signs: temperature, pulse, blood pressure and respirations are all taken into consideration, particularly in head injuries. A falling blood pressure and rising pulse indicate an unknown injury elsewhere in the body. (Head injuries alone rarely cause shock.)
b.   Observation of pupil size: a series of circular millimetre measures are used to establish the pupillary size.

Pupil reaction: using a bright light, the nurse should elicit whether the pupils are reacting or not. The non-reaction (and dilatation) of a pupil may indicate the presence of an expanding intracranial space-occupying lesion. It is not necessary to distinguish whether a pupil reacts briskly or slowly; only the presence of a reaction is important.

Limb movements: this part of the examination is required to differentiate limb movements in the presence of localised brain lesions. If the patient understands simple commands, he can be asked to lift his arms in the air or to demonstrate his hand grip in order that a comparison of both sides can be made. Failing this, the

PUPILS																																																		
L I M B	right	Size																																																	
		Reaction																																																	
	left	Size																																																	
		Reaction																																																	
A R M S	Normal power																																																		
	Mild weakness																																																		
	Severe weakness																																																		
	Spastic flexion																																																		
	Extension																																																		
	No response																																																		
MOVEMENT LEGS	Normal power																																																		
	Mild weakness																																																		
	Severe weakness																																																		
	Extension																																																		
	No response																																																		

+ reacts
— no reaction
c. eye closed

Record right (R) and left (L) separately if there is a difference between the two sides.

Fig. 2.4 Record of pupil size and reaction, and limb movements.

response can be assessed following painful stimulus. If the examiner feels that the response obtained from both limbs is within normal limits for that patient, then this is recorded as normal power. The keyword is comparison: one limb is compared with the other, which implies that if you judge one limb to be of normal power and the other mildly weak, then this is recorded as such. Likewise, if there is a large discrepancy in the strength of the limbs, this may be recorded as normal power on one side and a severe weakness on the other side. Recording differences between the two sides allows any discrepancies in limb movements to be graphically demonstrated. Spastic flexion, which is an abnormal reflex response, is included in this part of the chart. It is only applicable to the arms, which are stiff and slow moving, and indicates a degree of severe brain damage.

THE NEUROLOGICAL EXAMINATION

The description of the patient's symptoms and his medical and social background are recorded by the doctor when he interviews the patient and his relatives. It is interesting for the nurse to listen to the account, which will help her to understand how the information is elicited. An extensive, carefully taken history will give a good indication of the diagnosis. In epilepsy and other transient episodic disorders, where no signs are apparent on examination, the history is the only clue.

The patient's age and occupation are recorded. These give a guide to his level of intelligence and environmental factors which may have contributed to his illness, e.g. trauma or exposure to poisons, and the effect any disability may have on his future life, e.g. hemiplegia (paralysis of one side of the body), and which might prevent him returning to work.

The patient is asked if he is right or left handed so that the dominant cerebral hemisphere, which controls speech, is identified.

A detailed report of the nature, time or occurrence, and chronological relationship of symptoms to each other is sought and, as patients do not always volunteer information, specific questions are asked concerning the following.

Mental state. Has there been any change such as deterioration in memory, alteration in moods, drowsiness, episodes of unconsciousness or hallucinations?

Special senses. Has there been any visual impairment, e.g. double vision or loss of sight? Has there been any hearing defect, e.g. deafness or abnormal noises such as ringing in the ears? Has there been any giddiness? Has there been any disturbance of taste or smell?

Speech. Has there been any defect of speech?

Pain. Has there been any pain or headache?

Motor sense function. Has there been any abnormality in body movements, e.g. weakness or involuntary movements? Has there been any disorder of sensation, e.g. numbness or 'pins and needles'?

Bladder, bowel and sexual function. Has there been any impairment of bladder, bowel or sexual function?

Past history. A note is made of the patient's previous illnesses, hospital admissions and operations.

Family history. Enquiries are made concerning the family's medical history, with emphasis on neurological disorders, e.g. Huntington's chorea or muscular dystrophy. A very detailed family tree is sought.

Examination of the nervous system starts during the interview. The patient's mental state (whether he is alert or drowsy or confused), his mood (is it appropriate or is he unduly cheerful or depressed?), and his memory (can he remember the events in his illness or earlier life?) are noted. Any disorders of language (speech impairment or difficulty in comprehension of questions or instructions), gross weakness and involuntary movements will also become apparent. The examination proceeds as follows.

Assessment of intellectual function

The patient is asked the day, date, month, year, and to name the hospital and the queen. If he is unable to give the correct answers, there is obviously a severe disturbance of orientation.

Questions about general knowledge and current affairs are useful but may need to be adapted if the patient is a foreigner. All answers are considered in relation to the patient's educational background.

Problems of mental arithmetic can be used to detect mild intellectual deterioration, and one frequently used is the serial seven test. The patient is asked to subtract 7 from 100 and to continue subtracting 7 from the answer each time, i.e. 100–93–86–79. . . Normally this calculation can be performed accurately in less than one minute. Other tests include addition $(13+18+21)$ and multiplication (6×7) problems.

Mild memory impairment can be detected by giving the patient a simple name and address to repeat after 1, 5 and 15 minutes. The ability to repeat a series of numbers tests the immediate recall part of memory. Normally a group of six or seven figures can be remembered, and four or five in reverse.

In dementia (loss of intellectual capacity), the first function to be affected is the ability to learn new information. This is tested by asking the patient to repeat a complicated sentence, e.g. the Babcock sentence: 'The one thing a nation needs to be rich and great is a large secure supply of wood.' The examiner says the sentence and then the patient repeats it until he produces the correct version, which should be after fewer than five attempts.

Speech

Dysphonia is reduction in volume of speech due to disorder of the respiratory or laryngeal muscles, e.g. Parkinson's disease and myasthenia gravis. The voice is quiet or hoarse.

Dysarthria is difficulty in pronunciation and may be due to weakness or inco-ordination of the tongue and lips. In particular, it occurs in diseases of the cerebellum.

Dysphasia is a disorder of language. Difficulty in finding the correct words, i.e. expressive (motor) dysphasia, is tested by the examiner when he asks the patient to name a selection of common objects. Disturbances in writing, i.e. dysgraphia, also occur. A pencil and paper should be available to test for this.

Receptive (sensory) dysphasia is impairment in understanding of the spoken word. It may be tested by asking the patient to perform a simple test, e.g. 'put one hand on your head'. It is associated with difficulty in understanding the written word (*dyslexia*).

Perseveration is a tendency to repeat words or phrases. It may occur in patients with language disorders.

Agnosia

Agnosia is an uncommon disorder in which objects or sounds are not recognised. The inability to identify familiar objects by the sense of touch is termed *astereognosis*.

Apraxia

Apraxia is the inability to execute simple constructive movements, e.g. combing the hair or putting on a dressing gown, even though the muscles involved are functioning normally.

Spatial orientation and disorders of body image

A difficulty in visualising the relationship of different parts of an object leads to problems in drawing or copying geometrical figures, clocks or houses. The patient is often confused between the left and right sides of his body, and failure to appreciate where his limbs are, may contribute to dressing difficulties.

The last three types of disorders occur in lesions of the parietal lobes.

Examination of the cranial nerves (Fig. 2.5)

The olfactory nerve (I)

A selection of small bottles of aromatic substances is used to see if the patient can detect and distinguish the odours. Each nostril is tested separately.

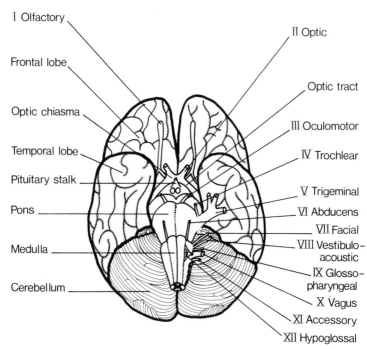

I Olfactory

II Optic

Frontal lobe

Optic tract

Optic chiasma

III Oculomotor

Temporal lobe

IV Trochlear

Pituitary stalk

V Trigeminal

Pons

VI Abducens

VII Facial

Medulla

VIII Vestibulo-
acoustic

IX Glosso-
pharyngeal

Cerebellum

X Vagus

XI Accessory

XII Hypoglossal

Fig. 2.5. *Inferior surface of the brain.*

The optic nerve (II)

Visual acuity. Each eye is tested for distance vision using a Snellen chart (letters on the wall 6 m away), and for near sight with test types (printed paragraphs of different sizes, e.g. the Jaeger chart) held in the patient's hand. If vision is severely reduced, then whether the patient is able to count fingers, observe hand movements, detect light or perceive nothing is recorded.

Visual fields (the area which the eye can see). Using a confrontation technique, the doctor is able to assess the patient's visual fields, and can compare them with his own. The patient is asked to cover one eye and with the other look at the doctor's opposite eye. Small objects (fingers or the coloured heads of pins) are moved towards the centre of the patient's gaze and he indicates when he first sees them. Four quadrants are tested, first in one eye and then in the other. Visual loss in any section is termed *hemianopia*, and when

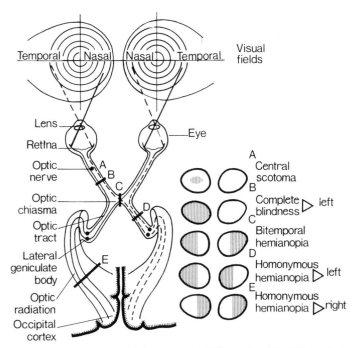

Fig. 2.6. *Visual pathways and defects in visual fields produced by different lesions.*

there is a complete or partial loss of the visual field affecting the nasal half of vision in one eye and the temporal half in the other, this is termed an *homonymous hemianopia* (Fig. 2.6). Two stimuli may be used on opposite sides of the field, and visual inattention is indicated when one is ignored.

A more detailed examination, using a perimeter or Bjerrum screen, may be performed if a defect is demonstrated by confrontation testing.

Fundi. The interior of the eye is examined using an ophthalmoscope (ophthalmoscopy). A complete view is obtained only when the head and eyes are kept perfectly still. Dilating drops should be very rarely used because they paralyse the pupil reactions for 24 hours and obscure the signs of neurological deterioration.

Abnormalities of the optic disc, e.g. papilloedema (swelling) or atrophy (pallor), are particularly important in neurology, as the former may indicate raised intracranial pressure and the latter may be an early sign of multiple sclerosis. Irregularities of the lens (e.g. cataract) or the retina (e.g. haemorrhage) are also noted.

The oculomotor (III), trochlear (IV) and abducent (VI) nerves

These nerves, which control eye movement, are tested together. The patient is asked to look up, down, to each side, and then up and down with the eyes deviated to the sides. Any defect of movement or complaint of double vision (diplopia) is noted. If nystagmus (jerking movements of the eyeballs) is seen, a description of its direction of movement (horizontal, vertical or rotary) and whether it is fine or coarse are noted.

The position of the upper eyelids is observed. Drooping is termed ptosis and elevation is known as lid retraction.

The pupils are examined with reference to their size, equality and regularity of outline. A pupil should react by constricting when a light is shone in the eye (direct) or in the other eye (consensual), and

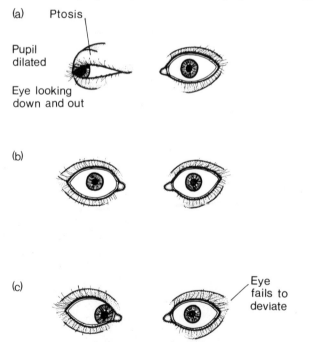

Fig. 2.7. (a) Oculomotor (IIIrd) cranial nerve lesion. (b) Abducent (VIth) cranial nerve lesion with eyes looking ahead. (c) Left abducent (VIth) cranial nerve lesion with eyes looking to the left.

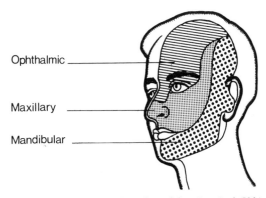

Fig. 2.8. *Areas supplied by the branches of the trigeminal (Vth) nerve.*

when the eyes converge to look at near objects, e.g. the tip of the nose.

A lesion affecting the oculomotor nerve produces a pupil which is dilated and unreactive, and because of muscle weakness the eye is deviated outwards and downwards and ptosis is marked (Fig. 2.7).

The trigeminal nerve (V) (Fig. 2.8)

The motor function. The muscles of the jaw are tested by asking the patient to clench his teeth so that the masseter muscle in the cheek and the temporalis muscle above the ear can be felt to contract. The jaw should open in the midline, and the patient ought to be able to withstand pressure from the examiner's hand to close it. The jaw jerk (reflex closure of the mouth on tapping the chin with a tendon hammer) is tested.

The sensory function. The three sensory branches are tested on either side using a pin and cotton-wool to touch the forehead, cheek and jaw. The corneal reflex (controlled by the ophthalmic division) is a blink in response to touching the cornea with a wisp of cotton-wool, which is introduced from the side after the patient has been asked to stare upwards.

The facial nerve (VII)

The motor function. The various groups of facial muscles are tested by asking the patient to frown, look surprised, close his eyes tightly, smile, whistle, and blow out his cheeks. All the movements should

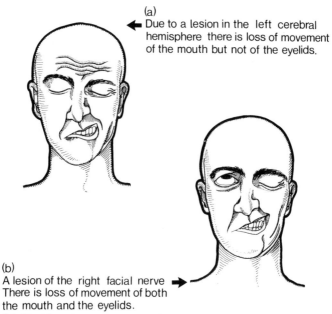

(a)
← Due to a lesion in the left cerebral hemisphere there is loss of movement of the mouth but not of the eyelids.

(b)
A lesion of the right facial nerve → There is loss of movement of both the mouth and the eyelids.

Fig. 2.9. *Facial weakness caused by (a) an upper motor neurone lesion, and (b) a lower motor neurone lesion.*

be symmetrical. Lesions of the cranial nerve or its nucleus in the brainstem, i.e. lower motor neurone lesion, affect all the muscles to cause lower and upper facial weakness (Fig. 2.9). Lesions in the cerebral cortex or internal capsule, i.e. upper motor neurone lesion, only produce a lower facial palsy, which is more apparent on voluntary than reflex movements. For example, there may be marked asymmetry when the patient is asked to show his gums, but when told a funny story his smile may be symmetrical. Tapping of the lips may cause pouting, and in some patients with severe degeneration of the brain, the introduction of an object between the lips will evoke sucking.

The sensory function. Taste is tested by putting drops of different solutions on the anterior part of the tongue. Saline (salt), syrup (sweet), quinine (bitter), and acetic acid (sour) test the four modalities. (A quantitative measurement of sensation can be made by passing a small electric current between electrodes on each side of the tongue and recording the threshold at which a metallic taste is perceived. This electrogustatometer is useful in assessing the progress of recovery in patients with Bell's palsy.)

The vestibulo-acoustic nerve (VIII)

The acoustic portion. On simple testing, the patient should be able to hear a whispered voice 50 cm from each ear. If hearing appears diminished, it is important to distinguish between deafness due to disease in the middle ear (conductive), which is very common, and that produced by a lesion of the inner ear or acoustic nerve (sensorineural), which may indicate important neurological disease.

Rinne's test. To test bone conduction of sound a vibrating tuning fork of 512 Hz (top C) is placed with its foot on the mastoid process. When it can no longer be heard, the open end is put by the auditory meatus to test air conduction. Normally, and in sensorineural deafness, the ringing is heard again, but in conductive deafness it is not. The contribution of the other ear is masked by using a clockwork noise box or merely by rubbing on the external meatus. (Quantitative measurements may be made by using electronically produced stimuli of different frequencies and intensities — audiometry.)

The vestibular portion. To determine vestibular function, caloric testing is performed (usually in an ear, nose and throat department). Each ear is irrigated in turn with warm water at 44°C (111°F) and cool water at 30°C (86°F), and the duration of the resultant nystagmus is noted. (This procedure often produces nausea in the patient.)

In coma of unknown cause, the ears may be irrigated with ice-cold water; deviation of the eyes to the side of irrigation will indicate that the brainstem is not involved.

The glossopharyngeal nerve (IX)

The sensation of the posterior part of the tongue and the pharynx is tested with an orange-stick. This should cause the patient to gag, i.e. to choke or splutter. The motor part of this reflex depends on the vagus nerve.

The vagus nerve (X)

Loss of the gag reflex necessitates withholding an oral diet. Difficulty in swallowing is termed dysphagia. The movements of the palate and uvula are noted when the patient says 'aah'. They should move upwards symmetrically. If the uvula is pulled to one side, there is weakness of the other. Hoarseness of the voice or a tendency to regurgitate fluids through the nose indicates weakness of the laryngeal and pharyngeal muscles.

The spinal accessory nerve (XI)

The patient is asked to shrug his shoulders to test the power of the trapezius muscles to raise them. Turning the head to one side is affected by the sternomastoid muscle of the opposite side, and resistance is provided by the examiner's hand on the chin.

The hypoglossal nerve (XII)

The patient is asked to open his mouth, and the tongue is inspected at rest. Any wasting and fasciculation (flickering contraction of muscle fibres without movement of the whole muscle) are noted. The patient is then requested to protrude his tongue; weakness of one side causes it to deviate in that direction.

Examination of the limbs

Initially, the limbs are inspected at rest. The characteristic flexed posture of the arm caused by an upper motor neurone lesion or a tremor of the hand due to Parkinson's disease may indicate the diagnosis. Any wasting or fasciculation of the muscles is noted. The girth of the limbs may be measured and compared with the normal side. In children apparent hypertrophy (enlargement) of muscles occurs in some forms of muscular dystrophy.

Tone of muscles is their resistance to passive movements, i.e. increased (spastic), normal, or decreased (flaccid). The patient is asked to relax each limb and let the doctor move the joints.

Power in all muscle groups of the arms and legs is tested by asking the patient to perform movements against the resistance of the examiner. The strength is compared between the opposite sides of the body. The pattern of weakness produced by upper motor neurone lesions, or damage to a single spinal nerve root or a peripheral nerve may be recognised.

Fine movements are examined by asking the patient to place the end of each finger in turn on the tip of the thumb on the same hand, or to make rapid 'piano playing' movements and to wriggle his toes quickly.

Co-ordination as a measure of cerebellar function is tested by the finger–nose–finger test, in which the patient is asked to place the tip of his index finger on his nose and then on the examiner's upheld finger and back to his nose several times. In the lower limbs the heel–knee–shin test is performed. The heel is placed on the opposite knee and moved down the shin to the ankle and back to the knee repeatedly.

In these tests both sides of the body are assessed. Speed and accuracy of movement and any tremor are noted.

The regularity of rapid alternating movements, e.g. tapping or twisting with each hand, is tested.

Tendon reflexes. A muscle is stretched by tapping its tendon with a tendon hammer, and the reflex contraction is observed. In a tense patient it may be difficult to elicit tendon reflexes because the muscles are already contracting. The patient is asked to clench his teeth or grip his hands and this contraction of other muscles often causes relaxation of the muscles being examined, thus allowing their reflexes to be demonstrated. This is called reinforcement.

In the upper limbs, the reflexes of the biceps, supinator and triceps muscles are tested; and in the lower limbs, tapping the patellar tendon produces reflex contraction of the quadriceps (knee jerk), and a smart tap on the Achilles tendon evokes contraction of the calf muscles (ankle jerk). The response is recorded as absent, diminished, normal or exaggerated, often abbreviated to 0, +, + + or + + + respectively.

When a muscle contracts and relaxes repeatedly, this is termed clonus, and it may be provoked by sustained stretching of a muscle, e.g. forcibly dorsiflexing (bending upwards) the ankle joint.

Superficial reflexes. The plantar response is obtained by firmly stroking, from the heel to the toes, the outer border of the sole of the foot with a sharp object, e.g. an orange-stick. The normal response is flexion of all toes. The abnormal (Babinski) reaction is spreading of the small toes and extension of the great toe. This occurs in lesions of the pyramidal tract anywhere between the cerebral cortex and the anterior horn cell, i.e. upper motor neurone lesion. The abdominal reflex is obtained by stroking the skin of the four quadrants of the abdomen with an orange-stick to provoke a contraction of the underlying muscles. The reflex is usually absent in upper motor neurone lesion.

Sensation. Information about different types of stimuli travel in different parts of the spinal cord. The patient's ability to appreciate various stimuli is tested at the extremities, and in some cases the trunk is also examined.

  a.   Pain sensation is tested by pin prick.
  b.   Temperature discrimination: the patient should be able to distinguish between tubes containing warm and cool water pressed onto the skin.
  c.   Light touch: the stimulus used is a piece of cotton-wool dabbed lightly onto the skin.
  d.   Joint position sense (proprioception): with the patient's eyes closed, the tip of one of his fingers or toes is moved and he is asked to indicate the direction of the movement, 'up' or 'down'.
  e.   Vibration sense: the footplate of a tuning fork vibrating at 128 Hz is placed on a bony protuberance (a knuckle, an ankle or a knee). The patient should be able to feel this at the fingers and toes, but such sensation is soon lost in peripheral neuropathy and lesions of the posterior column, e.g. due to multiple sclerosis.

Other forms of sensation sometimes tested include the ability to distinguish two close points, i.e. two-point discrimination; to recognise figures drawn on the skin, i.e. graphaesthesia; to identify (with eyes shut) objects such as a coin, key or india rubber, by their shape and feel when placed in the hand, i.e. stereognosis; and to detect two stimuli presented simultaneously to opposite sides of the body.

Examination of the head and trunk

The head

Any abnormalities in the size and shape of the head are noted. In infantile hydrocephalus, the vault of the skull will be too large for the face, the fontanelle bulges and percussion may produce a 'cracked pot' sound. The doctor examines the scalp for tenderness and places a stethoscope on the head so that any bruit due to an angioma may be detected.

The neck

Flexion of the neck is limited by tension of the muscles in meningitis and in some extrapyramidal disorders such as Parkinson's disease. Movements in other directions may be restricted and painful in degenerative conditions of the cervical spine.

The spine

The shape of the spine and its movements are inspected. Co-ordination and the ability to maintain a posture are tested by observing the patient sitting or standing. To distinguish between unsteadiness (ataxia) produced by lesions of the cerebellum and that caused by loss of joint position sense due to disorders of the peripheral nerves or spinal cord, Romberg's test is used.

Romberg's test. The patient is asked to stand still with his eyes open and feet together. He is then instructed to close his eyes and if, as occurs in loss of joint position sense, he sways and falls, the test is positive. (With his eyes open, the patient maintains his balance by looking at a stable object, but with the abolition of his sensory input there is inadequate information from the sense organs in the joints for the patient to remain upright.)

Examination of the gait (walking)

It is important to watch the patient walking, as many disorders may be diagnosed from abnormalities occurring in the gait. In Parkinson's disease the arms are held immobile by the side and the steps are short and shuffling, especially at first. The stiff swinging of a leg with scraping of the toe indicates an upper motor neurone lesion. A wide-based, irregular, unco-ordinated gait is due to cerebellar disease. High stepping is seen in patients with foot-drop. Stamping the feet is characteristic of tabes dorsalis.

Examination of the skin and joints

The state of skin may be an indicator of many disorders. In lesions of the autonomic nervous system, the ability to sweat is lost so the skin is dry. If sensation is disturbed, ulcers may have developed. Abnormal pigmentation of the skin is often associated with neurofibromas (tumours around nerves). Angiomas (arteriovenous malformations) of the skin and brain may occur together. Anaemia, apparent as skin pallor, is sometimes due to vitamin B_{12} deficiency, which can cause neurological disease.

The joints. Deformities and any limited range of movement of the joints (e.g. from rheumatoid arthritis) are noted because these may mimic weakness or pain due to neurological disease.

Examination of other systems

A complete examination of all the other systems is undertaken. The blood pressure and peripheral pulses are noted. A bruit may be heard over the carotid arteries when these are stenosed (narrowed). The heart and lungs are ausculated and the abdomen is felt for viscera and abnormal masses.

EQUIPMENT FOR THE NEUROLOGICAL EXAMINATION

The equipment (listed below) is usually kept in a large tray, which should be regularly checked and restocked when necessary.

Bottles containing test substances for smells — oil of cloves, peppermint, rosemary, asafoetida
Bottles containing test substances for taste — saline, syrup, quinine, and acetic acid
Ophthalmoscope
Reading chart
Pins with white heads and red heads
Torch with a bright light
Auriscope
Tuning forks 512 Hz, 128 Hz
Noise box
Tendon hammer

Dividers (for two-point discrimination)
Cotton-wool
Pins
Corked tubes for hot and cold water
Tape measure
Box of objects for testing dysphasia, e.g. comb, coin, penknife,
  pencil sharpener, safety pin, india rubber and key
Orange-sticks
Tongue spatula
Sphygmomanometer
Stethoscope

FURTHER READING

JONES, C. (1979) Glasgow Coma Scale. *American Journal of Nursing, 79*:9, 1551.
NIKAS, D.L. (ed.) (1982) *The Critically Ill Neurosurgical Patient,* p.1. Edinburgh:
  Churchill Livingstone.
TEASDALE, G.M. (1975) Acute impairment of brain function. 1. Assessing con-
  scious level. *Nursing Times, 71*:24, 914.
TEASDALE, G.M., GALBRAITH, S.L. & CLARKE, K.Y. (1975) Acute impair-
  ment of brain function. 2. Observation record chart. *Nursing Times, 71*:25, 972.
WALLECK, C.A. (1982) A neurologic assessment procedure that won't make you
  nervous. *Nursing (US), 12*:12, 50.

3 Investigations

Investigations are essential in order to confirm or reject a diagnosis made from the initial history. They also allow the surgeon to locate a particular lesion more accurately, thus providing greater safety when it comes to operation. It is instructive for the nurse to see the investigations being performed, and her first-hand knowledge of the procedure will help promote confidence in the enquiring patient and his relatives. Many neuroradiological procedures carry hazards in their performance, and any known possible complications should be fully explained to the patient. Some procedures require a consent for general anaesthesia, and this needs to be obtained by the doctor. In some remote cases, the investigative procedure can make the patient's condition worse, and this risk needs to be weighed against the outcome of the disease process itself.

The investigations of patients with suspected neurological disorders or injuries are many and varied and can involve many different departments within the hospital. The main investigations are as follows.

1. Neuroradiology
   Plain films of the skull, face, spine and chest
   Angiography
   Orbital venography
   Computerised transverse axial tomography
   Myelography
   Basal cisternography
   Air encephalography
   Ventriculography
   Echoencephalography
2. Ward level
   Lumbar puncture
3. Nuclear medicine
   Brain scanning (isotope)
4. Electrophysiology
   Electroencephalography
   Electromyography
5. Neuro-ophthalmology
   Visual field charting

RADIOLOGICAL INVESTIGATIONS

Plain radiography

The skull

X-rays of the skull are performed using various projections, the more common ones being lateral, anterior–posterior, and basal (submental vertical). Some more specialised views may also be employed.

Various features are noted in the interpretation of skull films. These would include the following.

1. Fractures: these may be linear, depressed or comminuted. They are invariably caused by trauma.
2. Alteration in bone density.
   a. Bone thinning may occur in patients with a metastatic tumour or generalised calcium deficiency.
   b. Bone thickening is found in Paget's disease or in hyperostosis.
3. Displacement of structures: the pineal gland is found in normal circumstances in the midline, but will be displaced in the presence of a space-occupying lesion.
4. Sutures: these may be found to be separated, as in hydrocephalus, or prematurely fused, as in craniosynostosis.
5. Intracranial air may be present when a patient sustains a basal skull fracture.

Tomography is a specialised technique in which the depth of projection is varied to define specific areas while blurring the rest of the skull bones. Tomography is important in defining very finite or early bone changes as they occur in:

a.   the pituitary fossa, when there may be asymmetrical erosion of the floor;
b.   the internal auditory meatus, where any increase in the diameter would be indicative of the presence of an acoustic neuroma.

The face

X-rays of the facial bones are performed when there is a history of trauma to the face or unexplained swelling of facial tissues following head injury. The views employed are usually occipital–frontal; occipital–mental, lateral, and soft tissue views. The purpose of these films is to define with greater accuracy the sites of fractures, fluid levels, or air in the sinuses. Orbital views will demonstrate fractures involving the walls, floor and roof of the orbits or any bone changes due to a tumour.

The spine

Projections used in spinal x-rays include anterior–posterior; lateral, and oblique. These views will demonstrate:

  a.   congenital defects, e.g. spina bifida;
  b.   degenerative changes;
  c.   bony erosions due to a primary tumour or tuberculosis;
  d.   widening of the foramina, as in neurofibroma;
  e.   fractures and dislocations.

The chest

A chest x-ray is routinely performed on most patients following admission to hospital. Many cerebral tumours are metastases, and carcinoma of the bronchus is a common primary site. The presence of a lesion may influence the management of the patient.

Angiography (arteriography)

Cerebral angiography

This is an x-ray examination in which the cerebral blood vessels are opacified by the injection of liquid contrast medium, e.g. Conray 280 or Hexabrix 320, and then demonstrated on serial x-ray films to show filling of the vessels.

A carotid angiogram is usually performed by injecting the contrast medium through a needle inserted percutaneously into the left or right carotid artery. This will show the anterior and middle cerebral arteries, i.e. the posterior part of the brain. Although the right or left vertebral artery can be injected in the neck, it is much more common for the femoral artery in the groin to be punctured

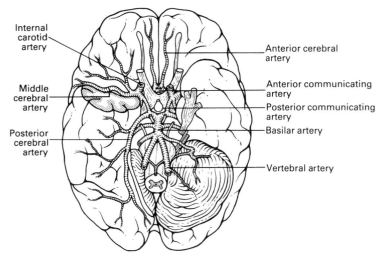

Internal carotid artery

Middle cerebral artery

Posterior cerebral artery

Anterior cerebral artery

Anterior communicating artery

Posterior communicating artery

Basilar artery

Vertebral artery

Fig. 3.1. *Circle of Willis.*

and a catheter threaded to the appropriate vessel. This approach may also be used for carotid angiograms (Fig. 3.1). The procedure is performed in the x-ray department using local or general anaesthesia. The patient lies supine on the x-ray table throughout the procedure. For each series of films, an injection of 8–10 ml, of contrast medium is given. Often, more than one artery is injected during the examination so that information about a large part of the brain and its blood supply can be obtained. When he removes the needle from the artery, the radiologist presses on the puncture site for five minutes so that the hole in the vessel seals itself and haemorrhage will not occur.

Related nursing skills. The following information should be passed on from the x-ray nurse to the nurse responsible for the patient's recovery: location of the puncture site(s), provisional diagnosis, and information on any special difficulties encountered during the procedure, e.g. a difficult cannulation.

During the recovery stage, the patient is nursed on his side and routine neurological observations are performed every 15 minutes initially, the frequency of observations being reduced according to the patient's recovery. Observation of the puncture site for swelling or bleeding is of vital importance, particularly in bilateral carotid punctures where the swelling could endanger the patient's airway.

Some risks are involved in cerebral angiography, and the nurse needs to be aware of these.

1. Reaction to the contrast medium. Some patients are allergic to iodine and collapse with low blood pressure (anaphylactic shock) when it is injected. This is usually apparent during the investigation, and despite treatment with large doses of intravenous hydrocortisone, the condition may prove fatal. The doctor should ask the patient if he is allergic to iodine before the procedure, and in doubtful cases a test dose must be given.
2. Injury to the arterial wall during the puncture may dislodge an atheromatous plaque or cause thrombosis in the vessel. Either may lead to cerebral infarction.
3. Injection of the contrast medium may provoke spasm of cerebral arteries, especially in patients with subarachnoid haemorrhage. The spasm may be so marked that cerebral infarction occurs.
4. Following the procedure, haemorrhage may occur at the puncture site. This is rarely severe, but a carotid haematoma can cause obstruction of the trachea.
5. Attempted puncture of the axillary artery may produce a pneumothorax which causes acute respiratory embarrassment.

In interpreting angiography films, the radiologist will check for:

a. displacement of vessels by a haematoma, cyst or tumour;
b. the sac of an aneurysm or the mass of vessels in an angioma (arterio-venous malformation);
c. abnormal vessels in a tumour which may demonstrate a pattern characteristic of a particular type of tumour;
d. absence of a vessel due to thrombosis; or narrowing due to atheroma.

Spinal angiography

The arterial supply of the spinal cord can be demonstrated by injecting contrast medium into the intercostal arteries. These arteries are studied individually by passing a catheter up from the femoral artery. Angiomas are well shown, and the technique is also useful in demonstrating the blood supply and site of other lesions.

The procedure may provoke ischaemia of the cord, giving rise to weakness of leg movements and disturbances of bladder function.

Orbital venography

Orbital venography involves injecting a small amount of a contrast medium into the appropriate frontal vein and then taking x-ray films to demonstrate the pattern of circulation around that area. This procedure, which is performed without any anaesthesia, is used in the investigation of suspected pituitary gland lesions, aneurysms, and tumours, and in the localisation of foreign bodies.

No special preparation is needed. Once the patient is positioned comfortably on the x-ray table, an elastic band is placed around the head, above the ears and just under the nose, and folded swabs are placed on either side of the nose to compress the facial veins against the maxillary bones. Two more elastic bands are placed around the head above the ears and extending around above both eyebrows, which has the effect of distending the frontal veins. A small intravenous cannula is inserted into the vein, and then more folded swabs are placed under the elastic bands above each eyebrow, thus compressing the supra-orbital veins but allowing contrast to flow into the ophthalmic veins. The contrast is then injected and the films taken.

Related nursing skills. No specific after care is usually needed, although some patients may develop a small haematoma.

Computerised transverse axial tomography (CT scan)

A relatively new neuroradiological investigation which has completely revolutionised the management of a wide spectrum of patients, this technique was invented by an English physicist called Godfrey Hounsfield and developed by the EMI Company (and thus often referred to as an EMI scan). It is not yet available in every neurological centre due to the high cost of the machinery, but the procedure's simplicity and comprehensive results will ensure that it will be in the future.

Head scanning

Computerised transverse axial tomography involves calculating the tissue density of an organ and, from the value obtained, a picture is subsequently produced. The patient lies supine on a motor-driven couch with his head pushed against a water-filled bag in the centre of the machine. The water bag reduces the layer of air as it moulds itself around the skull. For this investigation the patient must lie perfectly still as artefact distorts the final picture and makes inter-pretation difficult.

The vast majority of patients will co-operate in this procedure. However, elderly or confused patients and children may require a general anaesthetic. CT scanning is ideal for out-patient use.

A fan beam of x-rays is scanned across the patient's head in such a way that it enters edge on through a 1.3 cm thick plane taken transaxially through the patient. A bank of sodium iodide detectors on the other side of the patient picks up the intensity of the rays emerging, and these readings are then processed by computer. The mechanism is then rotated through 10°, the process repeated, and so on through 180°.

The absorption values of each square millimetre within the irra-diated slice are then calculated by a computer on a scale measured in Hounsfield units (HU) so that water = 0 HU, bone = 1000 HUs, grey matter = 34–44 HUs, white matter = 22–34 HUs, cerebro-spinal fluid = 0–8 HUs and air = 1000 HUs. Eventually a picture is built up which can be produced on a cathode ray tube screen, and then onto either an x-ray film or as a black and white photographic print.

One 'slice' takes only 60 seconds to perform and, depending on the number of 'slices' required in any one scan, the whole procedure can be done within 5–10 minutes. (Older machines may take up to one hour.) Previous limitations of this machine have now largely been eliminated, and further development is inevitable.

Contrast enhancement may be used in some cases. This involves giving the patient an intravenous injection of a contrast medium such as Conray or Urografin and then proceeding with the scan. Tumours, arterio-venous malformations and even large aneurysms will take up the contrast, and so will be highlighted on the films. Several scans may be performed to assess the progress of a disease, e.g. hydrocephalus.

Related nursing skills. Little or no nursing intervention is required. Patients should, of course, have the procedure explained to them, and any confused, frightened or very ill patients should have a nurse to supervise them. Patients having general anaesthetics require further care. They should be prepared for the general anaesthetic in the usual way, i.e. consent signed, identity bracelet in place, urine voided prior to transfer to the x-ray department, jewellery strapped and any dentures removed. A nurse must stay with the patient for the duration of the anaesthetic and scan, and should assist the anaesthetist where necessary. The after care requires the nurse to stay with the patient until he is fully awake, performing neurological observations and ensuring that he is comfortable.

Whole body scanning

A similar machine has been developed which permits CT scanning of the abdomen and thorax. However, there are limitations as to the fine detail in pictures of the spinal cord.

Myelography

A myelogram is a radiograph produced during an investigation in which a contrast medium is used to outline the spinal subarachnoid space, the spinal cord and its nerve roots. Two common contrast media in use are metrizamide (Amipaque), which is water soluble, and iophendylate (Myodil), which is an oil-based substance. Any irregularities in flow or temporary blocks may be demonstrated and could be indicative of a tumour or prolapsed intervertebral disc (Fig. 3.2).

Written consent should be obtained from the patient for the myelogram and a full explanation given by the doctor of the procedure involved. The skin over the lumbar spine may need to be shaved, and food and fluids are withheld for about 4 hours before the test because the tipping required to let the contrast medium flow along the spinal canal may cause regurgitation.

Following a lumbar puncture, the contrast medium is injected and the patient is then strapped to the x-ray table. Any cerebrospinal fluid removed is kept and sent for laboratory examination, where the cell count and glucose and protein estimations are performed. If Amipaque is used, the usual volume is 10 ml and it is necessary to keep the patient's head above the lumbo-sacral area in

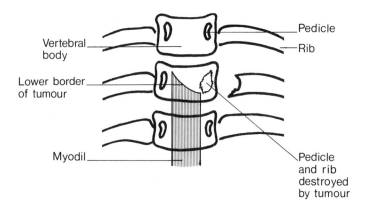

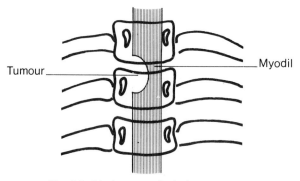

Fig. 3.2. *Myelograms of spinal tumours.*

order to avoid an irritant meningitis. If Myodil is used, the usual volume is 6–9 ml.

The patient is reassured that he will not fall, and the table is then tilted in various directions and at different angles. The contrast is visualised passing up and down the spinal canal by the radiologist using an image intensifier which produces a picture on a TV screen.

X-ray films are taken at various stages in the procedure and form a permanent record of the myelogram. (A nurse should stay with the patient throughout the procedure.) Once satisfactory results have been obtained, the contrast medium may be removed and the patient is returned to his own bed.

Related nursing skills

The pre-myelogram care involves obtaining a signed consent from the patient and ensuring that he has a proper understanding of what is to happen to him. The skin over the lumbo-sacral area may need to be shaved, and the patient is given an open-backed gown to wear. An opportunity to attend to toiletting needs should be provided immediately prior to transfer to the x-ray department.

A nurse should stay with the patient at all times during the myelogram. The patient will require reassurance that he will not fall when the table starts to tilt. The nurse can use this opportunity to gain the patient's confidence and thus ensure that he will co-operate with the investigation. It is essential that the nurse be aware of the potential dangers involved when a contrast medium is used. In a few rare cases some patients will have a reaction to the dye, and this can range from a mild rash to collapse of the cardiorespiratory system. The nurse will need to modify her actions, in a situation like this, as the need arises.

When the patient is transferred back to his bed, routine post-lumbar puncture nursing procedures should be adhered to:

a. the patient is nursed flat in bed for 24–48 hours;
b. fluid intake should be encouraged to replace lost fluids (200 ml hourly);
c. fluid output should be observed for retention of urine (which can occur when the spinal cord is compressed in the presence of a tumour);
d. puncture site must be checked for leakage;
e. analgesia should be given for back pain or headache.

Basal cisternography

A cisternal puncture is performed under either local anaesthetic or neurolept analgesia, and radiopaque dye is injected and x-ray films taken at several different projections to outline any filling defects within the basal cisterns.

The procedure is indicated in those patients requiring investigation of a suspected pituitary tumour or acoustic neuroma. Some centres advocate the use of a prophylactic anticonvulsant which is continued 24 hours after the x-ray.

Related nursing skills

Pre-x-ray:

1. The patient should be given an explanation as to what the investigation involves.
2. A consent should be obtained.

During x-ray:

1. The patient will require constant reassurance.
2. An ongoing check should be maintained of the patient's vital signs and colour. Any discomfort which the patient complains of should be reported immediately to the doctor.
3. The patient should not be left alone during the procedure.

Post-x-ray:

1. If metrizamide is used as a contrast medium, the patient is nursed sitting upright for 6–8 hours, to avoid an irritant meningitis.
2. The patient's level of consciousness, vital signs and colour should be closely monitored.
3. Fluids should be encouraged.
4. Analgesia or anti-emetics may be necessary and should be given as required.
5. Any chills or fever should be reported as these may indicate meningeal irritation or infection.

Lumbar air encephalography

Lumbar air encephalography, an investigation which uses air as a contrast medium to outline the intracranial subarachnoid space and ventricular system of the brain, is not performed nearly so frequently as it was at one time. It is an extremely unpleasant experience for a patient to endure, and has been replaced in many centres by the use of the CT scanner. The procedure involves the patient being strapped into a special chair following the induction of general anaesthesia. The patient's head is rested against the film holder and the neck flexed at the correct angle to encourage the air to enter the ventricular system. A lumbar puncture is performed with the patient in the sitting position and air is injected in various quantities in two or three stages. This is known as the fractional technique. A total of up to 50 ml of air may be injected. The contrast medium rises up the spinal canal to the cisterna magna, enters the fourth ventricle through the foramen of Magendie, passes upwards via the aqueduct into the third ventricle, and from there into the lateral ventricles. It also passes into the subarachnoid space outside the brain. X-rays are taken at various stages and from different directions. By tilting the head, the air can be manipulated as a bubble within the ventricular system. To make the air enter the temporal horns the patient has to be turned through a somersault.

Related nursing skills

The patient is prepared as for a general anaesthetic.

1. Written consent should be obtained from the patient.
2. The patient should be fasted for at least 8 hours prior to the x-ray being performed.
3. He should understand what is happening. (It is best to tell the patient that the procedure and its after-effects can be unpleasant.)
4. The patient should be bathed and a gown put on.
5. His identity bracelet should be checked.
6. Any dentures should be removed and jewellery strapped (a check list may be in use in some centres).
7. Case notes are taken by the nurse who accompanies the patient to the x-ray department.

During the procedure, a nurse should be present and the patient observed constantly for any signs of distress. The procedure should be stopped if necessary.

The nurse who transfers the patient following the procedure should be aware of the following information.

1. Which procedure was performed.
2. The provisional diagnosis.
3. Any special instructions, e.g. must the patient continue fasting for surgery.

The aftercare of the patient involves the following.

1. Close neurological observations. In patients with a space-occupying lesion, rapid deterioration may occur following air encephalography.

2. The patient should be nursed flat in bed with one pillow for 24–48 hours. Many patients take longer to recover and should be kept on bed rest as long as is necessary.
3. Fluid intake should be encouraged in order to replace cerebrospinal fluid that has been removed (200 ml/h).
4. Analgesia should be given for headache.
5. Puncture site should be observed for leakage.

Dangers of air encephalography. The dangers of air encephalography are as follows.

1. If the patient has a cerebral tumour, coning may occur. The removal of large quantities of cerebrospinal fluid may precipitate this emergency situation in the x-ray department or soon after the patient returns to the ward. Ventricular drainage via a burr hole must be instituted immediately.
2. Marked deterioration in patients with communicating hydrocephalus may ensue.
3. Profound postural hypotension and subsequent cerebral anoxia may develop because the patient is sitting while anaesthetised for about an hour.
4. A considerable rise in blood pressure with the danger of cerebral haemorrhage may be caused by injection of the air.

Ventriculography

Ventriculography is an investigation involving the injection of a contrast material (e.g. Myodil) into the ventricular system via a burr hole in an adult, or into the anterior fontanelle in an infant. This procedure is performed in order to localise tumours which may be pressing on, for example, one of the lateral ventricles and therefore causing it to appear misshapen on the x-ray film, or to check the patency of the ventricular system itself.

Ventriculography is yet another investigation which will increasingly be superseded by computerised axial tomography in time to come.

The patient is taken to theatre where a burr hole is performed on the non-dominant side, unless it is suspected that a tumour may be present on that side, and a catheter is inserted into the lateral ventricle. The catheter is secured in place, and the patient is taken to the x-ray department where the contrast medium is injected and the

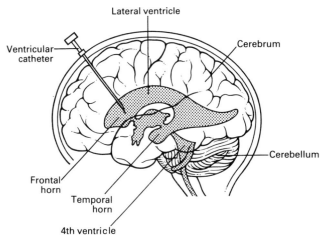

Fig. 3.3. *Side view of the head to demonstrate the position of a ventricular catheter.*

patient's position altered in order to demonstrate the part of the ventricular system to be examined. X-ray pictures are taken, as deemed appropriate by the radiologist (Fig. 3.3).

Related nursing skills

Pre-operative care. The patient is fasted for 6 hours; consent is obtained by the doctor, and the procedure explained to the patient. Immediately prior to transfer, the patient's identity bracelet is checked, dentures are removed and jewellery strapped in place. The patient should be allowed the opportunity to go to the toilet.

This procedure may be performed under local or general anaesthetic. Sometimes neurolept analgesia may be used in patients who will not tolerate the procedure under a local anaesthetic. This involves giving the patient a neurolept analgesic drug such as droperidol, with a narcotic analgesic such as phenoperidine. Alternative combinations of drugs may be used in some centres. Neurolept analgesia produces a quiet, inactive patient who will respond when spoken to.

After-care. The patient is kept on bedrest for 12–18 hours, and may require analgesia (for headache) and anti-emetics. Neurological observations are performed frequently, and the head of the bed may be slightly elevated. Oral fluids are encouraged to help replace the CSF removed during the investigation. An observant nurse will be aware of the complications and be ready to act as and when necessary. Complications can include headache, nausea and vomiting, seizures and postural hypotension due to sudden changes in position.

Echoencephalography

Harmless ultrasonic waves can be passed across the head by the use of a probe which is placed on the scalp above the ear. Certain structures, such as the third ventricle, will reflect a proportion of the waves back to a receiver, and these waves are then graphically displayed onto an oscilloscope screen for interpretation. Any displacement of well-known landmarks, especially midline structures, will be well demonstrated.

This investigation is extremely limited and is of little value when used on its own. It is, however, a simple procedure which can be performed on an out-patient basis, and is entirely risk free.

Little or no nursing intervention is required.

INVESTIGATION AT WARD LEVEL

Lumbar puncture

A lumbar puncture is the simplest and the commonest of the three methods used to gain access to the cerebrospinal fluid which circulates in the ventricles and the subarachnoid space. The other two approaches are into a ventricle (via the anterior fontanelle in an infant and a burr hole in an adult) and at cisterna magna level. Figure 3.4 illustrates the three puncture sites and shows how the spinal cord terminates at L1–2, thus enabling a lumbar puncture to be performed between L3 and L4 or L4 and L5 without cord damage.

The reasons for performing lumbar puncture can be divided into *diagnostic* and *therapeutic*.

Diagnostic

  1. To obtain a sample of cerebrospinal fluid in order to check its

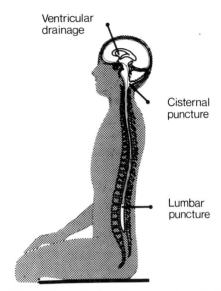

Fig. 3.4. *The three sites for obtaining cerebrospinal fluid.*

appearance. Normal CSF is crystal clear and so the patient who has a cloudy or blood-stained CSF requires further investigation and/or treatment. Sometimes blood may be old, and this presents as a yellowish tinge in the CSF: this is termed xanthachromia (see Table 3.1). Cerebrospinal fluid may be taken for biochemical and microscopic examination in the laboratory, and for culture and sensitivity studies.

2. To measure the pressure. (This is only feasible when the puncture site is at the same level as the head.) Space-occupying lesions and inflammatory disorders where the amount of CSF is increased, e.g. in meningitis, cause raised pressure. Blockage of the spinal subarachnoid space, e.g. by tumour, produces a low pressure, and Queckenstedt's test will confirm this.

3. To inject radiological contrast media, e.g. Myodil, for myelography, and air for air encephalography.

4. To introduce radioactive isotopes to study the CSF flow.

Therapeutic

1. Lumbar puncture facilitates the injection of drugs into the

Table 3.1 *The normal ranges of values and the abnormalities which may occur in lumbar puncture specimens in different diseases.*

Test	Normal	Abnormal
Colour	Crystal clear	(i) Blood-stained after a recent subarachnoid haemorrhage (ii) Yellow (xanthochromic due to blood pigments) (iii) Cloudy due to polymorphonuclear leucocytes in meningitis
Pressure	80 to 180 mm water	(i) Raised with a space-occupying lesion or infection (ii) Lowered in dehydration, e.g. diabetic coma
Cells (a) red blood (b) white blood (i) polymorphonuclear leucocytes (ii) lymphocytes 0 to 5 mm³	none	Present in subarachnoid haemorrhage (i) Polymorphonuclear leucocytes present (often thousands) in bacterial meningitis (ii) Excess lymphocytes (hundreds) in viral meningitis and tuberculous meningitis (iii) Malignant cells in carcinomatous meningitis
Protein	0·2 to 0·4 g/l	Moderate rise (0·5 to 1·0 g/l) in many neurological diseases. Marked rise (more than 1·5 g/l) in infective polyneuritis, with a neurofibroma, when the spinal canal is blocked by tumour.
Gamma globulin (IgG)	less than 13% of total protein	Raised in multiple sclerosis, neurosyphilis and immunological disease of the nervous system
Sugar	3·6 to 5·0 mmol	(i) Raised in diabetes mellitus (ii) Reduced (less than 2·9 mmol) in tuberculous and carcinomatous meningitis
Wassermann reaction	negative	Positive in neurosyphilis

subarachnoid space; this is termed an intrathecal injection. The most popular type of drug used in neurological departments is antibiotics, and they are specially formulated preparations which have no preservatives and are given in much lower doses. Anaesthetic drugs may be instilled intrathecally to induce spinal anaesthesia.

NB It is vital that the intrathecal form of the drug is used in this procedure; failure to use this form can result in the patient suffering seizures, severe headaches, a deterioration in conscious level and even death.

2. Occasionally, following surgery, a patient may develop a CSF leak through his craniotomy wound, and in some centres this would be treated by performing lumbar puncture and removing a quantity of CSF. This may be done for several successive days.

Contraindications to lumbar puncture

1. When it is suspected that the patient has raised intracranial pressure due to a space-occupying lesion: papilloedema suggests that the pressure is dangerously high, and removal of CSF by lumbar puncture may cause coning.
2. If there is infection of the vertebrae, lumbar puncture could spread this to the CSF.
3. Deformity of the vertebral column may deny access.

In (1) a ventricular tap is the only feasible approach, but in (2) and (3) the less involved technique of cisternal puncture may be used.

The procedure for a lumbar puncture

A full explanation is given to the patient. Any questions he may have should be answered by the doctor. The patient is asked if he wishes to empty his bladder and, if necessary, has his back shaved. He is then taken (where possible) to the treatment room.

The trolley should already be prepared with the following items.

A basic pack containing sterile swabs, gallipots, cotton-wool balls, drapes and forceps
Lumbar puncture needles (assorted sizes)
Spinal manometer

A three-way tap
Sterile surgeon's gloves
Scrubbing brush and sterile hand towel
Small cotton drapes (optional — many people use paper drape
 from basic pack)
Cleansing solution, e.g. Salvodil
Masks
5-ml syringe
Assorted sizes of needles
Local anaesthetic, e.g. 1% or 2% lignocaine
Adhesive plaster
Specimen containers
Request forms
Disposal bag

Additional items for intrathecal injection include: drugs to be injected, which must be suitable for intrathecal injection and be checked against the prescription chart and, finally, checked with the doctor before administration; syringe and needles; and a 0.22 μm-filter.

The usual position for lumbar puncture is with the patient lying on his side near the edge of the bed, i.e. the left lateral side, spine parallel to the edge of the bed, knees well flexed and head forward. This has the effect of opening the spaces between the vertebral spines. One pillow under the head and another separating the knees will prevent the shoulders and pelvis twisting (Fig. 3.5). When introducing contrast media, it is common to have the patient sitting upright.

A plastic and a cotton drawsheet should be placed beneath the patient to prevent a soiled bed, and with the puncture site exposed, he is then covered with a blanket. Once in this precarious position,

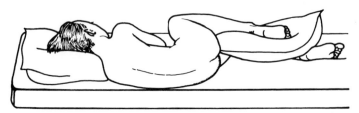

Fig. 3.5. *The usual position of the patient for lumbar puncture.*

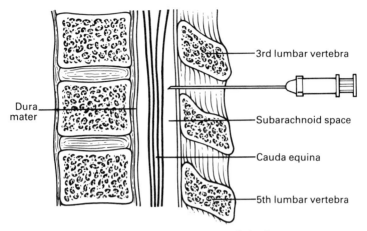

Fig. 3.6. *Lumbar puncture needle in situ.*

he must not be left unattended. The doctor scrubs up and dons sterile gloves and then organises his working surface. Forewarning the patient, he swabs a large area around the lumbar region with the cleansing lotion. He takes note of the previously marked puncture site and prepares to administer the local anaesthetic. It is drawn up after the doctor checks the contents of the vial with the nurse, and is then administered. It is important that the patient is told before the first injection is given as he may alter his position and so render the procedure more hazardous and difficult to perform.

Once the area is fully infiltrated, the doctor will select a lumbar puncture needle with which he will pierce the skin using a drilling action. The needle will pass through the intervertebral space until the resistance of the dura is overcome and the subarachnoid space is entered (Fig. 3.6). The stylet is removed and fluid drips out of the needle. If the pressure is to be measured, the manometer is attached and a note made of the reading (normal range, 80–160 mm).

Fluctuations of the pulse or respirations can be seen. To determine whether the CSF pathways are patent, a simple procedure (Queckenstedt's test) may be used. The venous return of the head is through the jugular veins and if one of these is compressed in the neck by the palm of the nurse's hand, blood is dammed back in the head and the pressure inside the skull rises. The cranial and spinal subarachnoid spaces communicate freely, so the pressure should rise in both and can be recorded on the manometer. If there is a spinal tumour, the rise in intracranial pressure is not transmitted to the lumbar region. The doctor will instruct the nurse when to compress each jugular vein, and the patient must be warned before a hand is placed on his neck as this action is naturally frightening.

False high pressure readings may be due to one of the following: a frightened patient who is very tense, or an obese patient who may be compressing his abdomen with his knees.

Samples are then obtained and deposited in the specimen jars, according to which tests are to be performed; 5–8 ml of CSF usually suffices. The specimen bottles should be labelled promptly and accurately, and then sent to the laboratory immediately (delay may affect the results).

The stylet is replaced halfway into the needle, which is then removed quickly and a small adhesive dressing or a dab of collodion is applied over the puncture site. After the patient has been settled comfortably and returned to the ward, the trolley is cleared away. The doctor records the procedure in the patient's case notes.

Related nursing skills

1. Set up trolley.
2. Shave the skin over the lumbo-sacral area (if required).
3. Ensure that the patient has the opportunity of emptying his bladder beforehand.
4. Reassure the patient. The nurse can allay the patient's anxiety by regarding the procedure as a routine investigation. A relaxed patient makes the procedure more tolerable for him and easier for the doctor to carry out.
5. Correctly position the patient in bed.
6. Observe the patient's colour, pulse and respirations during the procedure.
7. Assist the doctor as required.
8. Following completion of the procedure, remove soiled linen and make the patient comfortable.

Post-lumbar puncture care

1. The patient should be nursed flat with one pillow for 24 hours to avoid headache occurring.

2. Oral fluids should be encouraged to increase the speed of CSF replacement.
3. The puncture site should be checked frequently for leakage.
4. Routine neurological observations should be performed.
5. The following should be recorded in the nursing notes: the procedure performed; the time and date; the amount and character of fluid removed; the co-operation of the patient; and specimens sent to the laboratory.

Complications of lumbar puncture

1. Traumatic tap. The doctor may pierce a blood vessel on entry into the subarachnoid space. A traumatic tap is distinguished from a subarachnoid haemorrhage because the three consecutive specimens are not uniformly bloodstained.
2. Introduction of infection. It is very important that the doctor's and nurse's techniques are aseptic in order to avoid introducing infection which will cause meningitis.
3. Injury to the nerve roots in the spinal canal. Sometimes a patient complains of tingling or pain shooting down one leg. This is due to the tip of the needle touching a nerve root, and if he moves his leg or rolls over in bed, the root may be lacerated.
4. A CSF leak. Failure to seal the puncture site will allow CSF to escape slowly, thus exacerbating any headache the patient is suffering.
5. Coning. Patients with previously undiagnosed raised intracranial pressure due to a space-occupying lesion are liable to herniate following the removal of lumbar CSF. The removal of this fluid allows the brainstem to herniate down through the foramen magnum, often with fatal results.

Cisternal puncture

A cisternal puncture is very similar to a lumbar puncture in both procedure and aim, but it is performed at the level of the foramen magnum instead of below the termination of the spinal cord. This higher point of access to the subarachnoid space may be used to inject Myodil above a spinal tumour, or when a lumbar puncture is contraindicated.

The procedure is explained to the patient and the back of his head is shaved (Fig. 3.7) up to the occipital protuberance. The patient may be positioned on his side with his neck flexed and his head supported on one pillow, or he may be sat upright with his arms resting against pillows on a bed table.

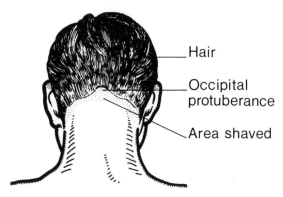

Fig. 3.7. *Area shaved for cisternal puncture.*

A cisternal puncture needle is slightly different from a lumbar puncture needle in that it has marks at centimetre intervals on the side. These are a safeguard against pushing the needle into the vital respiratory centre in the medulla.

NUCLEAR MEDICINE

Brain scanning

Brain scanning, a virtually hazard-free procedure, involves the use of radioactive tracers (isotopes), which are injected intravenously and the subsequent radioactivity detected with the use of a gamma camera. By far the most common isotope used is technetium-99m, which has a half-life of approximately 6 hours.

Before commencement of the investigation, the procedure is fully explained to the patient by the ward doctor. The patient, where applicable, is given an oral blocking dose of 400 mg of potassium perchlorate or, alternatively, 200 mg of sodium perchlorate intravenously, which has the effect of reducing the selective absorption of the isotope by the choroid plexus and therefore avoids the possibility of a false positive result.

After 30–60 minutes, the isotope, which is carried to the ward in a protective lead-lined box, is administered intravenously to the patient by the doctor wearing disposable gloves in order to avoid contamination. Once the isotope has circulated, which takes about 2 hours, the patient is taken to the department where his head is scanned using a gamma camera with back-up computer facilities. The camera has a battery of iodide detectors which monitor the radioactive distribution within the head. The scan is presented as a black dot density distribution on an x-ray film. Alternatively, some machinery produces a black and white photographic print. Abnormalities are detected by taking note of the changes in the radioactivity pattern from normal. The result is, in effect, a map of the blood–brain barrier and the cerebral blood volume. Isotope scanning is useful in the localisation of tumours, abscesses, subdural haematomas and infarctions.

The procedure can be performed with the patient either sitting on a chair or lying flat in bed. A complete scan, i.e. four views — anterior, posterior and right and left lateral — takes about 15 minutes to complete. It is a suitable investigation to perform on an out-patient basis.

Dynamic scans are performed immediately following the administration of the isotope, and the progress of the tracer can be followed through the blood vessels. An extension of dynamic scanning is the assessment of cerebral blood flow (CBF). Knowledge of CBF can help the surgeon to decide whether or not it is safe to operate, e.g. as in arterial spasm, following subarachnoid haemorrhage. Measurements of CBF during operation may indicate which surgical procedure is the safest or best, e.g. as in estimating the risk of cerebral ischaemia during carotid artery ligation.

Bone scanning can be performed, and this is useful in detecting metastases or infections within the bone structure. The isotope is tagged with a chemical which is phosphorus based and thus is taken up by the bone.

Nursing intervention in these procedures is minimal. No particular pre-scan preparation is required except to ensure that the patient has received his blocking dose. The patient should fully understand what is happening and may require a nurse to stay with him during the scan, to provide reassurance. In the post-scan period, local rules for handling radioactive materials should be observed.

Ventricular or CSF scanning

An isotope of indium with DTPA can be used to demonstrate the flow of CSF. It is administered via either a lumbar or cisternal puncture. The radioactive tracer flows with the CSF and within 12–24 hours should be detected within the area of the superior longitudinal sinus. The investigation is useful in detecting hydrocephalus.

In some centres, pledget tests are performed to confirm a CSF rhinorrhoea or otorrhoea. The isotope is administered via either the lumbar or cisternal puncture and, up to 30 minutes later, plugs are placed in either the patient's ears or nose. The plugs are left for 30 minutes to 1 hour and then removed, and the presence of any detectable radioactivity confirms that the patient has a CSF leak.

Related nursing skills

The patient needs to be prepared for a lumbar puncture and should receive adequate explanation and be kept informed of the progress of the procedure. Routine post-lumbar puncture nursing procedures should be applied.

ELECTROPHYSIOLOGICAL INVESTIGATIONS

Electroencephalography

An encephalogram is a graphic record of the electrical activity of the brain. Waves are picked up from the surface of the head, magnified and recorded on paper. Small electrodes, coated with silver chloride, are placed on the scalp in a standard pattern held by a hair net and/or collodion. The normal pattern of electrical activity can be recognised, and deviation from this suggests abnormal function of the brain cells, e.g. a tumour would be demonstrated as a localised abnormality which would be apparent throughout the recording.

Electroencephalography may be used as a routine screening test for suspected intracranial disease, but finds the following more specific applications in a neurological unit.

1. Diagnostic aid in patients with epilepsy.

2. Monitoring threatened cerebral ischaemia during trial occlusion of the carotid arteries.
3. Determining the probes in stereotaxic surgery.
4. Good localising value in patients with cerebral abscess.
5. In some countries, it may be used as an aid in determining cortical or brain death.

The greatest value of the electroencephalogram is in the diagnosis of epilepsy and distinguishing the different types. Sometimes the resting encephalogram is normal, and manoeuvres which increase the instability of the electrical activity are used. The simplest of these is hyperventilation, which reduces the carbon dioxide level; the patient is asked to breathe deeply for 3 minutes during the recording.

Flashing lights at varying frequencies precipitate petit mal in some susceptible patients. The instability is also greater when falling asleep or waking up. Sleep may be induced by an oral dose of diazepam (Valium) 20 mg, or an intravenous injection of methohexitone (Brietal). It should be noted that an encephalogram is not the ultimate proof that a person has epilepsy.

A sphenoidal electroencephalogram may be used in some cases of temporal lobe epilepsy where the abnormality is on the inferior surface of the brain and a long way from the electrodes on the scalp. Wire electrodes may be placed close to the undersurface of the skull through needles inserted into the cheeks (sphenoidal leads). These electrodes may detect discharges that were previously hidden.

Certain drugs, such as antidepressants or other psychotropic drugs, can interfere with the interpretation of the electroencephalogram, and these should be withheld for a period of 24 hours prior to the investigation.

Related nursing skills

For routine encephalography, the patient may sit in a comfortable chair or lie on a couch. In either instance, his neck must be supported with a pillow that does not disturb the electrodes. Prior to being sent to the department, the patient should have his hair washed and any hair oil removed. Women must remove any hairgrips. When the procedure is complete, any excess collodion is left to dry, then brushed out and the hair is washed again.

A sleeping encephalogram is more hazardous. Once the sedative is given, the patient should not be left alone. A consent is necessary and the patient is fasted for at least 4 hours prior to the investigation. Equipment including oral airways, suction and oxygen should be readily available in case the patient sustains a seizure while under sedation.

Electromyography

Muscle fibres generate electric currents which spread through the muscle causing contraction. This electrical activity can be detected by needle electrodes inserted into muscle; the potentials are amplified and displayed on a cathode ray oscilloscope. The experienced doctor can distinguish the normal patterns of an electromyogram from abnormalities due to disease of the muscle or of its nerve supply. The response of the muscle to electrical stimulation of its nerve supply can be observed and if the nerve is stimulated at two sites, the speed of conduction of the impulse — the motor conduction velocity (MCV) — can be calculated. In peripheral neuropathy, motor conduction velocity is reduced. Conduction in sensory nerves may also be studied. If electrodes are placed round a finger and electrical stimuli given, the electrical impulse may be recorded by electrodes placed over the nerve at the wrist, i.e. the sensory action potential (SAP).

Evoked potential measurements

An input is provided in the form of a stimulus, e.g. an auditory or visual stimulus, and with the use of strategically placed electrodes the conduction time (and therefore integrity of the nerve) is tested by comparing the patient's record with a normal one.

Visual evoked responses. The patient is asked to look at a flashing light or a patterned image, and electrodes are placed over the occipital lobes. Each eye is tested individually. Any delay in conduction time would indicate a lesion of the optic nerve, e.g. as found in multiple sclerosis.

Evoked potential audiometry. The stimulus consists of a clicking noise, and once again each ear is tested individually. The examination provides information about the integrity of the cochlea and auditory nerve.

Somatosensory cortical evoked potential. The electrodes are positioned over the sensory cortex and the stimulus is provided in the form of minute electrical charges. The examination commences with stimulation of the median nerve, and progresses at intervals following the route of the ascending sensory pathway to provide information about its integrity.

Little or no nursing intervention is required.

VISUAL FIELD CHARTING

Lesions can interfere with the normal field of vision by impinging on a section of the visual pathway, and these defects can be detected by the neuro-ophthalmologist using the direct confrontation method of visual field charting (Fig. 3.8). This type of testing requires the full co-operation of the patient.

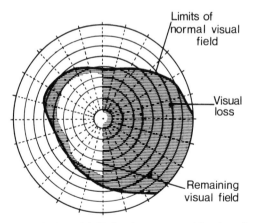

Fig. 3.8. *Visual field showing a temporal hemianopia.*

Bjerrum's screen

Bjerrum's screen is a large black screen with a white fixation point in the middle. The patient sits 2 m from it, covers one eye, and looks at the point. Any small defects in the visual field (including the normal blind spot) can be mapped out by moving an object on the end of a long black wand over the screen and noting when the patient can and cannot see it. Objects of different sizes (2 mm to 10 mm) and colours may be used, and both eyes are tested separately. This technique ascertains central vision close to the fixation point where acuity is greatest.

Lister's perimeter

This involves the patient resting his chin on the apparatus, and one eye is occluded. The patient is asked to fix his gaze on the central white spot of the metallic arc which is positioned exactly 330 mm away. The test disc is moved mechanically from the periphery inwards, and the patient indicates where the spot first comes into vision; this is repeated in eight different positions. The patient's chart is then compared to a normal record and any deficit noted.

FUTURE DEVELOPMENTS

Nuclear magnetic resonance scanning

Nuclear magnetic resonance (NMR) scanning is based on the principle that hydrogen nuclei will, in the presence of a static magnetic field, behave like small magnets and form up in the direction of the field, in this case in the long axis of the body. Radiofrequency magnetic pulses are added from a coil surrounding the patient and these are used to rotate the nuclear magnetisation, and the changing pattern produced will be received as an electrical signal in a receiver coil. By using different pulse sequences, an image is built up based on the local nuclear and molecular environment. The images produced are said to be clearer and better defined than those of the CT scan; however, NMR scanning is only available in a few centres. The research and development of suitable contrast material are being undertaken.

Little or no nursing intervention is needed. The patient lies flat on a table and is moved inside the machine as it operates. This may produce a feeling of claustrophobia, and the presence of a nurse is reassuring to these patients.

Positron emission tomography

Positron emission tomography (PET) studies areas of abnormal brain metabolism. A contrast medium, deoxyglucose with radioactive fluorine, is injected intravenously and the patient is then scanned. The scanner emits positrons which then collide with electrons to form photons. These are picked up by a bank of detectors and processed by computer to produce a colour map image of the glucose metabolism within the brain. Uses for this type of scan include preoperative localisation of epileptogenic cells, and postoperative assessment of cerebral blood flow.

Ambulatory electroencephalography

Ambulatory electroencephalography is performed using a portable recorder over a 24-hour period. Its use may be indicated in the diagnosis of petit mal or temporal lobe epilepsy, attacks of unknown origin, or of a possible hysterical overlay. Small electrodes are glued to the patient's scalp and the wires connected to a portable recorder attached to the patient's waistband or belt. The recording is made on a conventional cassette tape and this is analysed on a page mode display terminal at 60 times normal speed. A time clock is built into the machine, and the patient is provided with a device which he can easily operate, to indicate if he is about to have a seizure. This device 'marks' the tape and when it is played back it will automatically stop at this point and alert the examiner to an abnormal record. A disadvantage of this system is that if the patient is at home, a lot of artefact is produced, and only an experienced examiner can interpret the record. Patients are sometimes asked to keep written records of their activities throughout the recording period in an attempt to overcome this problem.

FURTHER READING

AMBROSE, J. (1973) Computerised transverse axial tomography 11. Clinical application. *British Journal of Radiology, 46*, 1023.

BURROWS, E.H. (1977) Myelography. *Nursing Mirror, 144*:11, 64.

BYDDER, G.M. (1983) Brain imaging by N.M.R. *The Practitioner, 227*:1377, 497.

CONWAY-RUTKOWSKI, B.L. (1982) *Carini and Owens' Neurological and Neurosurgical Nursing (PET)* 8th edn., p. 335. St Louis, Miss.: C.V. Mosby.

HOUNSFIELD, G.N. (1973) Computerised transverse axial tomography 1. Description of the system. *British Journal of Radiology, 46*, 1016.

KENDALL, B. (1979) A giant step forward in neurology (CAT scan). *Nursing Mirror, 148*:8, 35.

KREEL, L. (1976) Computerised trans-axial tomography. *Nursing Times, Key Clinical, 72*:25, 17.

MARSHALL, J. (1975) Radiology in the investigation of strokes. *Nursing Times, 71*:13, 511.

McMANUS, J.C. & HAUSMAN, K.A. (1982) Cerebrospinal fluid analysis. *Nursing (US), 23*:8, 43.

PETERSON, H.O. & KIEFFER, S.A. (1975) *Introduction to Neuroradiology*. London: Harper and Row.

ROBERTS, A. (1977) Lumbar puncture. *Nursing Times, Body Fluids Supplement, 73*,24.

SHEARER, D., COLLINS, B. & CREEL, D. (1975) Preparing a patient for EEG. *American Journal of Nursing, 75*:1, 62.

YOUNG, J.A. (1981) Head injuries-2. Advances in diagnostic equipment. *Nursing Times, 77*:19, 819.

4 Raised intracranial pressure

Many nurses will encounter patients suffering from the effects of raised intracranial pressure, and in order to understand why this happens we must first look at the processes involved in maintaining a normal intracranial pressure.

Contained within the very rigid skull, there are non-compressible contents, i.e. brain tissue, blood and cerebrospinal fluid. These three constituents maintain the delicate balance of intracranial pressure and are constantly fluctuating in response to activity such as coughing, which raises intracranial pressure, and standing, which lowers intracranial pressure. These are normal responses. An increase in any one of the constituents will mean that, following an initial period of compensation, one of the other two must decrease its volume in order to accommodate any alteration in intracranial content. If this is not possible, intracranial pressure will rise.

It should be noted that certain compensatory mechanisms are present when intracranial pressure rises: the blood volume will decrease and the CSF becomes displaced, but only to a limited extent. There are four stages in the process.

1. *The compensation phase*: no rise is seen in intracranial pressure, and conscious level is unaltered.
2. *The early phase of reversible decompensation*: a small increase in the mass lesion will result in a large rise in intracranial pressure. Some downward changes may be noted in the patient's conscious level.
3. *The late phase of reversible decompensation*: intracranial pressure continues to rise and the patient shows a marked deterioration in conscious level. The respiratory pattern will also change. The situation is rapidly being approached where the intracranial pressure will equal the systolic blood pressure, which will result in vasomotor paralysis leading to cessation of cerebral blood flow and death.
4. *The irreversible decompensation phase*: a continuation of phase 3, the patient will continue to deteriorate and die.

CAUSES OF RAISED INTRACRANIAL PRESSURE

Blood

Hypoxia → increased blood flow → raised intracranial pressure.

Carbon dioxide retention → dilatation of the cerebral veins → increased blood flow → raised intracranial pressure.

Cerebrospinal fluid

Increased production, e.g. due to a tumour in the choroid plexus → raised intracranial pressure.

Decreased absorption, as can be caused by the presence of blood within the CSF, prevents adequate absorption in the arachnoid villi → raised intracranial pressure.

Blockage of the pathway, e.g. by a tumour → enlargement of the ventricles (hydrocephalus) → raised intracranial pressure.

Brain

Space-occupying lesion, e.g. tumour or haematoma → raised intracranial pressure.

Cerebral oedema, caused by an increase in extracellular or intracellular water → raised intracranial pressure.

SYMPTOMS OF RAISED INTRACRANIAL PRESSURE

Headache

Headache occurs in the early morning, and may even waken the patient from sleep, and disappears within an hour or so. The headache is usually described as throbbing and is aggravated by coughing or stooping.

Vomiting

Vomiting may occur in conjunction with the early morning headache and may be projectile.

SIGNS OF RAISED INTRACRANIAL PRESSURE

Papilloedema

Raised intracranial pressure is transmitted down the optic nerve and, when the fundus is examined using an ophthalmoscope, the clinician may see a swollen nerve head. Papilloedema, however, only occurs after the intracranial pressure has reached fairly high levels, and may not even be present in some patients, while in others it may be the first sign.

The three classical signs and symptoms of raised intracranial pressure must be observed within the context of the patient as a whole. Other signs and symptoms must be taken into account, and these may include:

- *a.* a deteriorating conscious level;
- *b.* changes in pupillary responses;
- *c.* a change in the respiratory pattern;
- *d.* bradycardia which is full and bounding;
- *e.* a compensatory rise in blood pressure followed by a fall;
- *f.* an elevation in body temperature.

Coning

If there is an expanding lesion such as a tumour, abscess, haematoma (extra- or intracerebral) or the dilated ventricles in hydrocephalus, then the pressure is not equally raised in all compartments, and attempts are made to compensate by a shift of cerebral tissue from one area to another. This is called herniation. When herniation of tissue from a high- to a low-pressure compartment occurs, it is said that a pressure cone has been formed, and the process is often referred to as 'coning'.

Supratentorial cone or uncal herniation

When a space-occupying lesion is situated above the tentorium, the uncus (which is the lowest and most medial part of the temporal lobe) is forced down through the hiatus (opening) in the tentorium on one or both sides (Fig. 4.1). This hole is occupied by the upper brainstem, which contains the reticular activating system (on which consciousness depends) and the oculomotor nuclei. The uncal

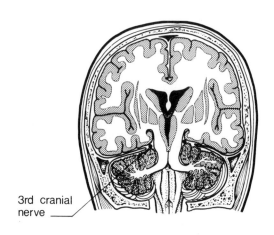

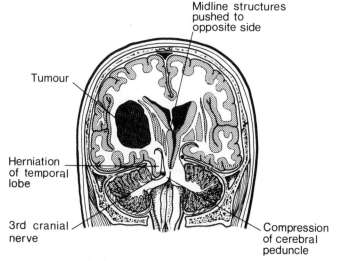

Fig. 4.1. *Normal coronal section and a section showing herniation of part of the temporal lobe through the tentorium due to a mass in the cerebral hemisphere (tentorial cone).*

(a)

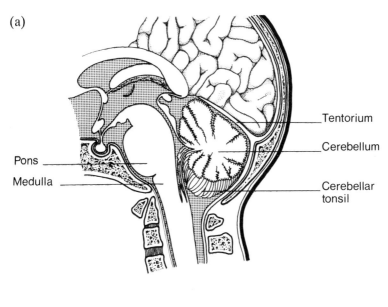

Tentorium

Cerebellum

Pons

Medulla

Cerebellar tonsil

(b)

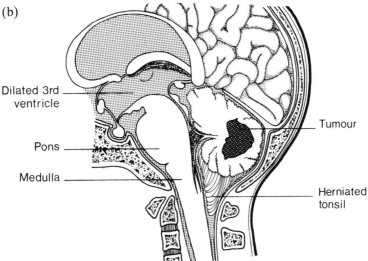

Dilated 3rd ventricle

Pons

Medulla

Tumour

Herniated tonsil

Fig. 4.2. *(a) Normal posterior fossa and comparative study, with (b) herniation of cerebellar tonsils through the foramen magnum due to a cerebellar tumour (cerebellar, infra-tentorial or foramen magnum cone).*

hernia compresses the brainstem producing depressed consciousness and disturbance of eye movement.

Cerebellar or infratentorial cone

A lesion in the posterior fossa tends to press the lowest parts of the
cerebellum, i.e. the tonsils, downwards into the foramen magnum,
where they compress the medulla oblongata which has also been
pushed down (Fig. 4.2). This structure contains the vital respiratory
centre, and continuous compression leads to Cheyne–Stokes respiration, followed by irregular shallow respirations, and finally
cessation of breathing. The speed at which either of these processes
occurs depends on the nature and site of the causative lesion. An
acute extradural haemorrhage from a torn middle meningeal artery
complicating a fracture of the temporal bone, may lead to a supratentorial coning in a few hours, while a cerebellar abscess associated
with an ear disease may take days or weeks, a chronic subdural
haematoma weeks or months, and a slow-growing tumour years.
However, alteration of pressure gradients between compartments,
as when cerebrospinal fluid is removed at lumbar puncture, may
rapidly change the progress and precipitate an acute pressure cone.
The final stages often occur very quickly, and the nurse can frequently avert a fatal outcome by recognising and reporting the early
signs. It is essential to keep detailed records of the level of consciousness and of the respiratory pattern, as well as of the pulse and
blood pressure, for small, but progressive, changes are the initial
warning signals.

Conscious level

A change in the level of consciousness is an important early indication of brainstem distortion. If a standardised conscious level charting system (e.g. the Glasgow Coma Scale) is used, this allows easier
and safer observation of the patient.

Pupils

Normally, the pupils are equal in size and react briskly to light. The
oculomotor (third cranial) nerve is compressed at the tentorial

hiatus when an uncal herniation occurs, leading to the pupil on this side enlarging and slowing in its response to light. In time, the pupil becomes widely dilated and unreactive (fixed). Any variation in pupil size or reaction should be reported at once.

Pulse rate and blood pressure

Raised intracranial pressure causes a slowing of the pulse and a rise in blood pressure during the late stages.

Respiratory pattern

Brainstem distortion may produce several types of disturbance in the breathing pattern, including hyperventilation and Cheyne–Stokes respirations, but the most serious is respiratory depression, as this indicates a medullary compression and can lead to respiratory arrest. Slowing of respirations to 10/minute (or below) should be reported.

All these parameters are measured at frequent intervals, as dictated by the patient's condition. It is on the nurse's observancy that the doctor, who is not with the patient constantly, will rely. Any changes should be reported immediately and recorded in the patient's charts.

FACTORS AFFECTING INTRACRANIAL PRESSURE

1. Inadequate ventilation resulting in an increase in the arterial PCO_2 and a lowered PO_2 will vasodilate the cerebral blood vessels, and this will result in an increase in cerebral blood volume, leading to a rise in intracranial pressure.
2. A rise in intra-abdominal and/or intrathoracic pressure caused by coughing or sneezing is transmitted to the spinal subarachnoid space and subsequently to the veins that communicate with the dural venous sinus. The cranial vault is impeded and intracranial pressure rises.
3. Certain drugs may raise intracranial pressure, for example halothane.

MEASURING INTRACRANIAL PRESSURE

Many patients with raised intracranial pressure will require some form of monitoring, and this may be performed for any one of several reasons.

1. To monitor a deteriorating conscious level when neurological assessment is impeded, and thus to guide diagnosis and effective treatment.
2. To monitor treatment in order to gauge its effectiveness.
3. To aid diagnosis in patients suffering from hydrocephalus.
4. To act as an early warning system in the detection of complications such as a recollected haematoma following craniotomy.
5. To act as a prognostic guide to outcome.

Methods of measuring intracranial pressure

There are several ways that this can be done, but all current methods rely on the principle of transmitting the level of pressure from within the patient's head onto a chart recorder with the use of a catheter, a transducer and a pen recorder or oscilloscope.

Intraventricular measurements

A burr hole is made and a catheter is placed in the lateral ventricle. This is then connected via fluid-filled tubing to a transducer, located either on a bedside stand or strapped to the patient's head. It is important that the transducer is level with the tip of the ventricular catheter before a true reading is taken, and all subsequent readings must be taken in the same way.

The transducer converts the pressure within the tubing to an electrical signal, which is then relayed to a pen recorder or oscilloscope for interpretation. The disadvantage of this method is the small risk of infection and the even more rare problem of haemorrhage along the catheter tract. An advantage is that there is access to the ventricular system so that cerebrospinal fluid can be drained off or fluid added if necessary. Radiological procedures can also be performed at no further inconvenience to the patient.

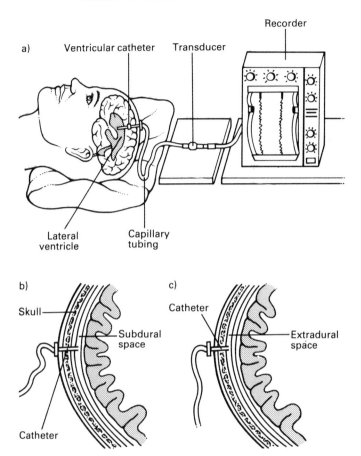

Fig. 4.3. *(a) Intraventricular pressure monitoring. (b) Subdural pressure monitoring. (c) Extradural pressure monitoring.*

Subdural or subarachnoid measurements

This method involves making a hole in the skull with a special drill and then fitting a hollow metal bolt which reaches into the subdural space. The bolt is connected up to the transducer and recorder as described in the first method. The risk of infection is about the same, although the catheter tract haemorrhage problem is eliminated.

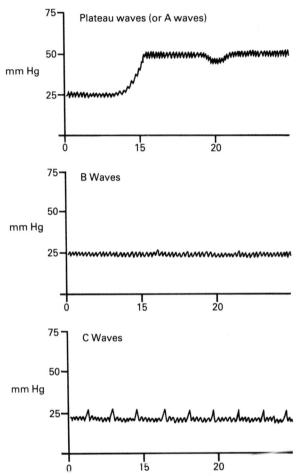

Fig. 4.4. *Intracranial pressure waveforms (time scale in minutes).*

Extradural measurements

The least used of all, this involves inserting a transducer into the skull so that a diaphragm is applied to the dura and recordings can be made of the extradural space pressure (Fig. 4.3).

Interpretation of intracranial pressure monitoring

The most significant finding when a patient's intracranial pressure is monitored is a high reading. Significant values vary, but most agree that any reading over 15 mmHg is abnormal; levels over 20 mmHg are moderately elevated, and sustained levels over 40 mmHg are severely elevated. High readings may be present for several hours in some patients, but in others transient wave-like elevations may present themselves.

There are three main types of wave (Fig. 4.4).

1. A waves or plateau waves: the name is derived from the shape of the wave (see Fig. 4.4). These rise suddenly from an already elevated baseline and last 5–20 minutes before falling, sometimes to below the original level. They often reach up over 50 mmHg at their peak and can cause cerebral ischaemia and brain damage, and so are of important clinical significance.
2. B waves: these are sharp, rhythmic oscillations which occur every $\frac{1}{2}$–2 minutes and peak at between 10 and 15 mmHg. They are usually seen in relation to a fluctuating respiratory pattern such as Cheyne–Stokes respirations.
3. C waves: these occur more frequently, at 4–8 per minute, and may raise the intracranial pressure by 20 mmHg. They correspond to changes in blood pressure and are of little significance.

Related nursing skills

Patients undergoing intracranial pressure monitoring need to be nursed on bedrest until the monitoring is completed. Many of these patients have an impaired conscious level and will require the necessary specialised care in addition to the following special considerations.

1. To enable accurate readings to be performed, the transducer must be level with the tip of the ventricular catheter. The transducer will either be strapped to the patient's head or attached to a bedside stand; in the latter case the height of the bed stand will need to be altered in relation to the position of the patient's head.
2. A high degree of asepsis must be maintained. Any breaches in the system should be investigated immediately, and the doctor informed.
3. The nurse must be familiar with the machinery and feel confident using it.

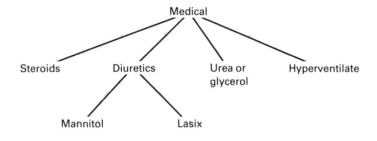

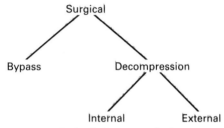

Fig. 4.5. *Medical and surgical methods of alleviating raised intracranial pressure.*

4. Any variations in the readings must be recorded. The best place to do this is on the patient's coma chart, and the readings must be taken each time the level of consciousness is assessed.

The following should be reported.

1. Any rise in intracranial pressure or the presence of A, B or C waves.
2. The loss of the pulsatile waveform.

Each time an artefact is produced on the recording paper following such manoeuvres as suctioning or moving the patient, the nurse should indicate this on the paper.

MANAGEMENT OF PATIENTS
WITH RAISED INTRACRANIAL PRESSURE

This is determined by the patient's general condition and what may be causing the raised pressure. The aim is to reduce the increased pressure and prevent it from recurring. In the acute stages, where the patient presents with a sudden rise (as found with a head injury), immediate relief of pressure is vital and the cause must be treated, e.g. evacuation of the offending haematoma.

The patient with a slowly rising intracranial pressure, such as may be caused by a slow-growing tumour, would require the appropriate investigations and treatment in order to deal with the problem. A patient presenting with papilloedema would be admitted urgently to hospital, as this usually indicates a fairly high level of pressure.

Alleviation of raised intracranial pressure can be divided into medical and surgical means (Fig. 4.5).

Medical management

Steroids

Many tumours, and all inflammatory lesions of the brain, produce cerebral oedema with swelling of the brain, and an increase in intracranial pressure. Steroids reduce this oedema, and the most potent is dexamethasone, which may be given orally, intramuscularly or intravenously in doses up to 4 mg, 6-hourly, with an initial dose of 8–16 mg. There is a delay of about 12 hours before the effects become apparent. When the treatment is prolonged, the side-effects of steroid medication may occur, and the nurse must be alert for these.

Diuretics

If a major pressure cone is formed with loss of consciousness or cessation of respirations, more rapid treatment is required. Intravenous therapy with diuretic drugs produces systemic and cerebral dehydration, resulting in lowering of the intracranial pressure. Frusemide (Lasix) 20–80 mg intravenously may be adequate treatment, but a hypertonic solution of mannitol is more effective. Mannitol is an osmotic diuretic, being excreted unchanged by the kidneys and taking with it sufficient water from the body to be diluted in the urine. The water is absorbed from the brain into the blood and then excreted with the mannitol. A common dose is 20 g, which is given as 100 ml of a 20% solution, or 200 ml of a 10% solution infused over 15 minutes.

Speed is essential in the institution of treatment because brain cells suffer irreversible damage within 3–4 minutes if the oxygen supply is cut off by respiratory or cardiac arrest or severe local compression. The action of mannitol is often rapid and dramatic. The heart beat returns, breathing recommences, the conscious level lightens, and the patient may become sufficiently alert to ask what has been happening. A large quantity of urine is voided, often more than 1 litre, and in order that this may be measured accurately, a urethral catheter is inserted when the mannitol infusion commences. The nurse should note the amount of urine passed and check whether analysis of the urine is required.

The above description has been for mannitol, but a concentrated solution of urea may be used in exactly the same way. In less urgent situations, the doctor may prescribe a dose of glycerol to be given via a nasogastric tube. Although rapid action may be accompanied by a dramatic improvement, the results are not always successful. The effect of diuretic drugs on raised intracranial pressure is temporary, and if the patient is to benefit, alternative methods of controlling the pressure are needed.

Controlled ventilation

Patients with raised intracranial pressure may benefit from controlled ventilation. This is indicated where control and protection of the airway are required in order to maintain adequate arterial blood gases. If blood gases are not maintained within normal limits, the patient will become hypoxic and/or hypercarbic, which will lead to a raised intracranial pressure and brain damage. Patients with chest injuries, hypo- or hyperventilatory breathing patterns, or persistent hyperpyrexia (which increases oxygen demand) are suitable candidates for ventilation.

Related nursing skills

When administering steroids, it is important that the correct drugs are given at the correct times and in the proper dosage. Any sudden cessation of treatment should be avoided. The administration of steroids can present some problems for the patient: steroids can alter the salt and water balance within the cells, resulting in retention which produces peripheral oedema and hypertension. Serum potassium levels may fall, causing a generalised weakness. Some patients may complain of gastric irritation, and some centres advocate the use of a prophylactic histamine-receptor antagonist, e.g. cimetidine (Tagamet).

Mannitol should be kept where it is readily available, and each nurse in the ward should be aware of its location. Mannitol comes in two concentrations — 10% and 20% — and the nurse must ascertain, from the doctor, which one to use. The usual dosage for an adult of average build would be 100 ml of the 20% solution infused over 15 minutes. Before administering the fluid, the nurse should check that crystallisation has not occurred (due to prolonged storage) and that the i.v. site is satisfactory. If a urinary catheter is not already in place, one should be inserted, and urinary output monitored closely.

If the patient requires artificial ventilation, a high degree of nursing is necessary, and the patient should be transferred to an intensive care area.

The following points need to be considered.

1. Two-hourly positional changes.
2. Light support for the patient's head and neck.
3. Two-hourly eye and oral hygiene.
4. Four-hourly urinary catheter care.
5. Supervision of i.v. fluids, including the cannula site and infusion rate.
6. Frequent vital signs and neurological observations.
7. Frequent checks to ascertain the safe working of the ventilator.
8. Sedation administered as required.

Surgical management

The patient may need to have a by-pass procedure performed in order to drain off excess cerebrospinal fluid. In an acute situation, this can be done on a temporary basis by the insertion, via a burr hole, of a small catheter into one of the lateral ventricles. The catheter is then connected up to a drainage bottle, which acts as an overflow mechanism provided the bottle is maintained at the correct height at the head of the bed. If the intracranial pressure does rise again, the excess cerebrospinal fluid flows out into the bottle, thereby maintaining the pressure at a tolerable level.

The system does have disadvantages.

1. An infection risk for the patient. The cranium acts as a protective barrier for the brain against infection. If a ventricular catheter is inserted, then the protective barrier is penetrated and an entry is provided for harmful bacteria. This infection

risk can be reduced by the use of a strict aseptic technique while inserting the catheter, and later as little manipulation of the system as is possible.
2. The bottle may move from its original predetermined level. If it is lowered, too much cerebrospinal fluid is drained off, and the patient will suffer low-pressure headaches; if it is raised, any effective drainage will cease and intracranial pressure will rise.

In patients with an inoperable lesion, a more permanent by-pass arrangement may be required. This would mean inserting a ventriculo-peritoneal or ventriculo-atrial shunt, a system which would draw off excess cerebrospinal fluid from the ventricles and deposit it in either the peritoneum or atrium for dispersal (see Chapter 21).

Other forms of treatment which may be used on a palliative basis include radiotherapy and an internal or external decompression. An internal decompression is produced by removing part of the tumour or by sacrificing healthy brain tissue, and an external decompression involves excision of part of the bony skull and dura. Both allow an extra outlet for the expanding lesion, though neither is performed now as frequently as in the past.

Related nursing skills

Patients requiring external ventricular drainage need special consideration when it comes to nursing. Bed rest is essential, and indeed some of these patients will have a compromised conscious level. The following points need to be observed.

1. A strict aseptic technique should be employed at all times. The dressing over the catheter site should be kept clean and dry. If the drainage bottle becomes disconnected, the tubing should be clamped as near to the skull as possible and the contaminated equipment discarded. The doctor should be informed and a new system set up.
2. The drainage must be kept at the prescribed level: if raised, the system will cease to work and intracranial pressure will continue to rise; if lowered, too much cerebrospinal fluid will drain off and the patient will suffer low-pressure headaches.
3. The drainage bottle and tubing will have to be changed every 24 hours, preferably at the same time each day, using an

aseptic technique. The amount of cerebrospinal fluid drained should be noted, and specimens sent to the laboratory for a cell count, measurement of sugar and protein levels, and detection of organisms, culture and sensitivity.

4. Care must be taken to ensure that there are no kinks in the tubing.
5. Tubing must be clamped temporarily when moving the patient onto a trolley.
6. Any variation in the colour of the cerebrospinal fluid (e.g. is it cloudy or bloodstained?) should be reported. (Normal cerebrospinal fluid is crystal clear.)

FURTHER READING

ALLAN, D. (1982) Nursing aspects of artificial ventilation. *Nursing Times, 78*:24, 1006.

BRUYA, M.A. (1981) Planned periods of rest in the ICU: Nursing care activities and ICP. *Journal of Neurosurgical Nursing, 13*:4, 184.

HICKEY, J.V. (1982) *Clinical Practice of Neurological and Neurosurgical Nursing*, p. 143. Philadelphia: Lippincott.

HILLMAN, K.M. (1982) Intracranial pressure monitoring. *Nursing Times, 78*:24, 1003.

JENNET, W.B. & TEASDALE, G.M. (1981) *Management of Head Injuries*, p. 122. Philadelphia: F.A. Davis.

JONES, C.C. & CRAYARD, C.H. (1982) Care of ICP monitoring devices: a nursing responsibility. *Journal of Neurosurgical Nursing, 14*:5, 255.

MILLER, J.D. (1978) Intracranial pressure monitoring. *British Journal of Hospital Medicine, 19*:5, 497.

MITCHELL, P.H., OZUNA, J. & LIPE, H.P. (1981) Moving the patient in bed: effects on ICP. *Nursing Research, 30*:4, 212.

NIKAS, D.L. (ed.) (1982) *The Critically Ill Neurosurgical Patient*, p. 29. Edinburgh: Churchill Livingstone.

SAUL, T.G. & DUCKER, T.B. (1982) Effect of intracranial pressure monitoring and aggressive treatment on mortality in severe head injury. *Journal of Neurosurgery, 56*, 498.

YOUNG, M.S. (1981) Understanding the signs of intracranial pressure: a bedside guide. *Nursing (US), 11*:2, 59.

5 Head injury

Head injuries are the most important cause of death and severe disability in young adults. Over 100 000 people are admitted each year to hospital in the UK with head injuries, although less than 5% of that total are transferred to a regional neurosurgical unit. Approximately 1500 brain-damaged survivors are discharged annually from hospital, with an average age of 30, of which half will never work again.

CAUSES OF HEAD INJURY

The most common cause of blunt or non-penetrating head injury in the UK is road traffic accidents. Other causes include industrial accidents and, within large inner-city areas, assault. Sport contributes to the total, the most hazardous being horse-riding.

Penetrating head injuries occur when the head is struck by a sharp object which produces an entry wound and, in some cases, an exit, e.g. as caused by a bullet. This type of injury is not common in civilian life.

A head injury is termed open if the brain is exposed, i.e. when the scalp, the skull and the dura have been breached. If the scalp is not damaged over the site of the fracture, this is a closed injury. The distinction is important to remember; in an open-wound injury the patient is at a far greater risk of infection.

It should be noted that defining injuries as open or closed does not necessarily indicate the severity of the injury. If a skull fracture is noted, this would imply that the injury has been moderately severe; but many patients with a simple fracture recover, whilst other patients die as a direct result of head injury without a skull fracture or even a mark on their scalp.

MECHANISMS OF HEAD INJURY

An impact injury will produce certain forces within the head which are detrimental to the patient. These forces are interrelated and occur, simultaneously or in rapid succession, to varying degrees. It

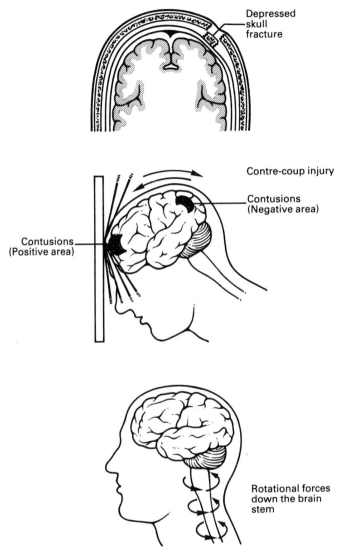

Fig. 5.1. *Mechanisms of head injury.*

should be noted that the most important factor governing the outcome of a head injury is the damage sustained by the brain, most of it occurring at the moment of impact (Fig. 5.1).

Skull deformation

In skull deformation, there is distortion of the contour of the skull, often resulting in a fracture.

Acceleration–deceleration injury

At impact, e.g. to the frontal area, the head moves backwards, and because of the small time delay involved in the movement of the brain itself, the frontal lobes strike the frontal bones, and at the same time a negative pressure area is set up at the occipital horns, producing maximum stress forces on the brain tissue. Direct injury at the point of impact and directly opposite is termed contre coup.

Rotational forces

These are the most devastating. The rotatory forces cause shear strains on nerve fibres and can extend in a spiral fashion all the way down the brainstem, causing severe damage and even death.

EFFECTS OF HEAD INJURY

The effects of head injury may be viewed in relation to the structures involved: the scalp, the skull, and the brain.

Injury to the scalp

Injury to the scalp is frightening to both the patient and bystanders because the skin overlying the head is very vascular and haemorrhage may be profuse. The scalp is not very significant in the consideration of injury, and even very large lacerations heal easily because of the excellent blood supply.

Injury to the skull

Trauma to the skull varies with the type of injury. The violence following a blunt injury is widely distributed throughout the vault of the cranium, which, because of its egg shape, is able to withstand considerable forces. If the stress is too great, distortion occurs and the bone fractures. The crack may be a simple linear fracture at the site of the trauma, or there may be extensive radiating fissures. These tend to spread into the base of the skull because this part is weakened by perforations and air sinuses.

The bones of the skull have a very rich blood supply and any fracture heals quickly, therefore its presence is not an important factor in the management of the patient. However, there are three exceptions to this: fractures involving air sinuses, depressed fractures, and fractures overlying the middle meningeal artery.

Fractures involving the air sinuses

A fracture which involves the frontal or paranasal sinuses can be recognised by the escape of clear fluid from the nose (cerebrospinal fluid rhinorrhoea), which to the patient tastes salty and, on testing with a dipstick reagent, is found to contain glucose. The significance of this leak is that infection can spread from the nose to the intracranial cavity. Treatment consists of antibiotic therapy and sitting upright in bed to reduce the intracranial pressure and diminish the leak. The patient is instructed to wipe the drip with tissues and not to blow his nose, as this might force infected fluid from the sinuses back into the subarachnoid space. Some patients may have a cerebrospinal fluid otorrhoea (a leak via the ear). If the leak does not cease spontaneously, the dural defect can be repaired with a patch of fascia, which is usually taken from the thigh.

Depressed fractures

A depressed fracture occurs when a fragment of bone has been forced below the normal level of the skull, and in an adult this is usually associated with tearing of the dura and laceration of the brain tissue. If the scalp is damaged at this site, infection can be introduced into the brain. Early operation is performed to elevate the piece of bone, to repair the defect in the dura and to excise any dead or infected brain tissue to reduce the risk of post-traumatic epilepsy.

Fractures overlying the middle meningeal artery

If the artery ruptures, blood spills into the extradural space causing an extradural haematoma.

Injury to the brain

In minor head injuries, distortion of the brain tissue ensues and there may be shearing forces between the grey and white matter. This stretching of the nerve fibres causes interruption of their function, and the brainstem reticular formation, which is responsible for consciousness, is particularly affected. The resultant episode of unconsciousness is brief and followed by a swift and complete recovery. This disturbance of nerve function is known as concussion and although it appears to be reversible (as there is no residual neurological deficit), some permanent damage must be sustained in view of the fact that repeated minor head injuries, as received by boxers, can lead to dementia.

More severe trauma to the head produces bruising of the brain tissue (cerebral contusions) in the areas of direct and contre coup injury, and the distortion of the brainstem is more marked. Consciousness is lost for a much longer period and when it is regained there may be a neurological deficit, e.g. a hemiparesis, but this often improves rapidly and the patient recovers fully. These patients require effective supportive management during the initial phase following injury, if deterioration of their conscious level is to be avoided. Once deterioration occurs, the options available for treatment are considerably narrowed.

In the most serious head injuries, coma may persist for days, weeks, months or indefinitely. The brain may also sustain a laceration which causes a permanent neurological deficit. Although this is usually at the site of direct injury, a tear of the temporal lobe by the sharp sphenoid ridge may be produced by a contre coup injury lesion. If a fracture of the base of the skull lacerates the brainstem, death or permanent coma follows.

The primary brain damage attributable to the head injury occurs at the moment of impact and, provided that complications can be avoided, the course is usually one of recovery.

The medical and nursing management is formulated around keeping the patient alive during the period of coma and maintaining close observation for any deterioration. Another objective is to minimise the degree of secondary brain damage which may occur. Improved care has been achieved through the creation of specialised neurosurgical intensive care areas and with it the effective use of modern technology, e.g. computerised monitoring, the advent of the CT scan, a greater awareness of the complications that can occur and, most importantly, the role played by the properly trained neurosurgical nurse.

Anyone sustaining a blow to the head should be examined by a doctor. If there is any evidence of brain damage or skull fracture, the patient should be detained in hospital for 24 hours in order that 2-hourly conscious level observations may be performed, to detect any early complications.

EARLY COMPLICATIONS OF HEAD INJURY

Intracranial haemorrhage, when it occurs, presents a major problem for the patient. Each of the haematomas is given its name according to its location.

Extradural haematoma (Fig. 5.2)

This occurs most commonly when the temporal bone is fractured, causing rupture of the middle meningeal artery, which subsequently bleeds into the extradural space. The haematoma continues to expand, and then at a critical point in any given time scale, the patient's conscious level will deteriorate. A typical history consists of a blow to the head followed by a temporary loss of consciousness; the patient then displays a lucid interval which may last for several hours, followed by another loss of consciousness. The patient may complain of headaches, become very drowsy, have seizures, develop a hemiparesis and a dilated ipsilateral pupil which subse-

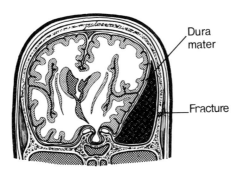

Fig. 5.2. *Extradural haematoma.*

quently becomes fixed. If these signs are not recognised and no treatment is initiated, the patient will become apnoeic and die.

Once a diagnosis of extradural haematoma is suspected, emergency treatment should be instituted. A temporal burr hole should be performed on the same side as the fixed pupil in order to relieve the damaging raised intracranial pressure and evacuate the haematoma. This can be a potentially life-saving procedure and should be performed without delay. This may mean doing it in the anaesthetic room or even the ward or, if a neurosurgeon is not available, the task may fall to a general surgeon.

An infusion of mannitol will provide a temporary relief of symptoms, thus facilitating transfer to a regional centre for treatment.

Subdural haematoma (Fig. 5.3)

This occurs as a result of bleeding into the subdural space between the dura and the arachnoid. There are three types:

   a.   acute, producing symptoms within 24–48 hours;
   b.   subacute, producing symptoms within 2 days to 2 weeks; and
   c.   chronic, producing symptoms during or beyond the 6th week.

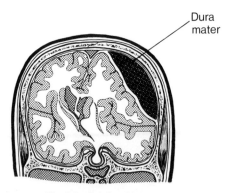

Dura
mater

Fig. 5.3. *Subdural haematoma.*

Acute subdural haematoma

The source of bleeding is usually from the small vessels bridging the subdural space and/or the contused areas of the brain. Compression signs develop rapidly and the patient quickly loses consciousness. (There is no lucid interval.) The patient may also develop an ipsilateral fixed dilated pupil and hemiplegia. Diagnosis is by CT scanning, followed by craniotomy and removal of the haematoma.

Subacute subdural haematoma

The presenting picture is rather less dramatic than the acute haematoma. Generally, failure to improve at the expected rate rather than sudden deterioration is more common. Treatment consists of bilateral burr holes and irrigation with saline to evacuate the clot.

Chronic subdural haematoma

This often occurs in the elderly, and the accident which produces it is so trivial that mention of it is entirely omitted by the patient and his relatives. As people age, the brain tends to shrink a little, thus allowing it to move more freely within the skull. A slight blow to the head may be sufficient to rupture some of the small veins which cross from the cerebral cortex to the dura.

The bleeding into the subdural space continues slowly and a haematoma forms. The patient, however, is frequently without symptoms for several days or even weeks.

With the clot gradually increasing in size, the patient begins to complain of headaches, or members of his family notice he is more forgetful or slightly confused. A hemiparesis develops, and fits sometimes occur. Characteristically the signs fluctuate. The patient may be drowsy and confused one day, fully alert and orientated the next day, only to deteriorate again.

A shift in the pineal gland, indicating a space-occupying lesion, may be noted on plain skull x-ray and confirmed by CT scanning. Burr holes are made in the parietal and frontal regions, sometimes on both sides as bilateral haematomas are not infrequent.

Recovery of full consciousness is often dramatic following aspiration of the haematoma(s), but fluid tends to re-collect in the evacuated cavity. This produces recurrence of the drowsiness and hemiparesis, and repeated subdural taps may be necessary. This procedure can be performed in the ward treatment room. Following infiltration of the area with local anaesthetic, a needle is introduced through the scalp into the burr hole and the fluid is aspirated. A note is made of the amount of fluid withdrawn and some may be sent to the bacteriology laboratory for examination. If repeated aspirations fail to prevent the reaccumulation of fluid, a craniotomy is performed and the capsule of the haematoma removed.

Intracerebral haematoma (Fig. 5.4)

This occurs as a result of bleeding into the cerebral tissues, usually from an associated laceration or contusion, and can be found deep within the hemisphere. The patient will present with a clear history of moderate to severe head injury, rapid loss of consciousness, an ipsilateral fixed dilated pupil, and a contralateral hemiplegia. Diagnosis is confirmed with CT scanning or angiogram, and treatment is surgical evacuation of the haematoma. Many of these patients do not recover, and those who do often have a neurological deficit.

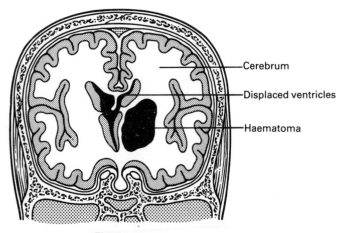

Fig. 5.4. *Intracerebral haematoma.*

Infantile subdural haematoma

Infantile subdural haematomas from head injury at birth are usually encountered in boys and develop within 6 months. Vomiting, irritability, convulsions and an increase in head circumference indicate that intracranial pressure is rising, and bilateral subdural taps via the anterior fontanelle are the means of confirming the diagnosis and treating the condition. Following several daily aspirations, bilateral temporal burr holes are performed to check for (and, if present, remove) the tough membrane that often forms and if left could impede cerebral growth.

Some children receive their head injury as a result of a non-accidental blow to the head, and in these cases the doctor will contact a paediatrician and the social worker in order that they may investigate the circumstances surrounding the incident.

Traumatic subarachnoid haemorrhage

An intraventricular haemorrhage can occur following severe head trauma, although this is rare. Conservative management is employed, the patient being nursed as a 'subarachnoid' patient.

Related nursing skills

Care of the conscious patient

On the ward, the routine preparations to receive an emergency admission are undertaken, including a check that clean airways, oxygen and suction are available. The patient is nursed flat, with one pillow, in an easily observable bed, to which cot sides can be attached. Too often, a quiet patient is left, only for it to be discovered that he is not asleep but deeply unconscious.

The nurse will record frequent neurological observations, having explained to the patient that these are a necessary disturbance. She should check whether fluid and food are to be withheld for the first few hours in case the patient deteriorates and requires an emergency operation.

The majority of patients with head injuries make a rapid recovery and can be sent home the following day with instructions to rest for two or three days before returning to work. If a fracture of the skull has caused some subarachnoid bleeding, a persistent headache will be complained of, and these patients are kept on bed rest and given analgesia until the headache has resolved. They are then rapidly mobilised and discharged.

Following a head injury, restlessness and confusion often produce problems in the nursing care of the patient. There are three common factors contributing to the confusional state:

a. headache due to subarachnoid haemorrhage;
b. intoxication by alcohol or drugs;

c.   amnesia: loss of memory is a constant accompaniment of
head injury and is due to the disturbance in cerebral function.
Retrograde amnesia, i.e. loss of memory for events prior to
the accident, varies from a few seconds to several years and is
longer in the more serious head injuries. The duration is also
influenced by other factors, especially intoxication by alcohol.
The period of post-traumatic amnesia, i.e. loss of memory for
occurrences after the accident, also depends on the severity
of the injury. A patient may have recovered consciousness
and yet still be in the stage of post-traumatic amnesia. He
may not remember the accident or what has been said to him
a few minutes before, and this transitional period between
coma and complete recovery of all intellectual faculties is
when confusion is most marked.

Care of the restless patient

Apart from cerebral irritation, the patient may be restless because
of pain due to other injuries or a distended bladder. In the latter
instance, recognition and relief of the discomfort may settle the
patient (no analgesic that will alter the patient's conscious level
must be used), but if he is passing through the post-head injury
confusional state, the condition will only abate with time.

The patient's agitation may be demonstrated by repeated
attempts to climb out of bed, throwing objects, shouting and resist-
ing any interference. If the nurse cannot persuade the patient to
take oral fluids (at least 2000 ml every 24 hours), the doctor may
decide that the patient should be fed either via a nasogastric tube or
by intravenous infusion. If the patient is still very noisy, he may be
moved into a side ward to avoid disturbing other patients. Sedatives
are withheld because they can mask neurological deterioration. The
doctor should decide at what stage some form of restraint should be
used.

Restraining a patient inhibits his freedom and may add to his
agitation. However, it is occasionally necessary as a protection for
the patient and others. Great care is needed in the choice of
restraints and how they are applied, to avoid permanent physical
damage to the limbs. Splinting the elbows so that both arms are
extended should prevent the patient from removing an infusion into
a vein in either arm or a nasogastric tube. In addition, bandaging of

the hands is required in aggressive patients. A soft roll of cotton-wool or bandage should be placed in the palm of the hand so that the fingers grip it. If the fingernails are long, the roll must be large enough to prevent them digging into the hand. The fists should be covered with padding and then wrapped with bandages. The end-result should resemble boxing gloves. Although the bandages need to be firm, they must not be tightly applied for fear of restricting the blood supply to the hand. The bandages must be removed for 5 minutes at least four times each day to examine the hands, to wash them and to move the fingers freely.

If the patient's arm movements need curbing, then using one of the patented wrist restraints is the safest way to do this. When the wrists are fixed in this way, the patient cannot turn, and so his pressure points must be treated 2-hourly. It is unnecessary and very dangerous to restrain a paralysed limb.

The nurse attending the confused patient should remain calm, answer his repeated questions rationally, and not be offended by his insulting behaviour. This behaviour is a reflection of the patient's cerebral illness, and the nurse's tranquillity often has a soothing effect.

Even the most gentle-mannered patients become abusive and restless during confusional states, and this is very distressing to their relatives, as is the sight of the patient strapped down in bed. The nurse must always explain the situation before the relatives visit the patient, and her sympathy will help them through this difficult stage in the patient's recovery.

Care of the unconscious patient

The following is a checklist of care.

Maintain a clear airway
Regular assessment of conscious level
Monitor vital signs
Protect the patient from injury
Position limbs carefully
Passive range of movement exercises
Eye care
Oral hygiene
Care of bladder and bowels, including care of the urinary catheter

Supervise i.v. fluids and site

Aspirate the nasogastric tube 2-hourly or, alternatively, administer feeds

Observe for cerebrospinal fluid leak

Psychological care of the patient and relatives

Elaboration of these points can be found in Chapter 6.

LATE COMPLICATIONS OF HEAD INJURIES

Post-concussional syndrome

This is the term applied to the symptoms of dizziness, headache and lack of concentration frequently encountered after minor head injuries. These features usually resolve within a few weeks, but in some patients they continue and increase in severity. An understanding approach usually reduces the duration of the disorder.

Anosmia

Anosmia (loss of the sense of smell) is caused when the violent movement of the brain inside the skull tears the olfactory nerves. The disability, which rarely recovers, is enhanced by the associated loss of taste discrimination (only the crude flavours of salt, sweet, sour and bitter are preserved). Apart from being denied the enjoyment of food and the appreciation of pleasant odours, e.g. flowers, the patient is at risk from his inability to perceive warning smells, e.g. escaping gas or burning.

Blindness

On rare occasions, a fragment damages the optic nerve and, because this cannot regenerate, the loss of vision is permanent.

Meningitis

When the brain is exposed to pathogenic organisms following an open, depressed or sinus fracture, prompt treatment with antibiotics is usually sufficient to prevent an intracranial infection. However, meningitis may develop, the patient being photophobic, restless, irritable, pyrexial and complaining of head and neck ache.

Epilepsy

Post-traumatic epilepsy occurs if the cerebral cortex has been damaged, and is therefore encountered after cerebral laceration and depressed fractures, especially if the wound has been infected. Prophylactic anticonvulsant therapy (phenobarbitone and phenytoin) is given following surgical excision of these injuries, but otherwise it is withheld unless the patient has a fit (i.e. up to one year after the accident).

Mental changes

Mental changes are common after severe head injuries. Personality disorders usually show as irritability and aggressiveness, and there may be general intellectual impairment. The patient is often unable to return to his job, and may be incapable of keeping a new, less taxing one. Some patients turn to alcohol as a relief from their frustration.

Dementia

Bleeding into the subarachnoid space gives rise to adhesions which obstruct the flow of cerebrospinal fluid. This progressive communicating hydrocephalus may cause dementia and is considered in any patient who deteriorates slowly over weeks or months, especially if incontinence is a prominent feature.

Frequent minor head injuries produce dementia, as in professional boxers who become 'punch drunk'. A patient who sustains a second head injury may be left with a severe disability although his recovery after the first episode was good. It would appear, therefore, that the brain damage caused by head injuries is cumulative.

Skull defects

Skull defects may be seen in patients with penetrating head wounds when portions of the skull are destroyed by the missile. If possible, the deficit should be repaired to restore the protective covering to the brain, but the operation is not performed until all the scalp wounds have healed completely and there is no evidence of infection. The defect may be closed by a metal or a plastic plate or by strips of bone taken from another part of the body.

FURTHER READING

ADAMS, J.H. (1976) Patients who talk and die after a non-missile head injury. *Nursing Mirror, 142*:17, 55.

ADELSTEIN, W. (1980) Chronic subdurals. *Journal of Neurosurgical Nursing, 12*:1, 36.

BOWERS, S.A. & MARSHALL, L.F. (1982) Severe head injury, current treatment and research. *Journal of Neurosurgical Nursing, 14*:5, 210.

CONNELLY, R. & ZEWE, G.E. (1981) Update: Head injuries. *Journal of Neurosurgical Nursing, 13*:4, 195.

COPPLESTONE, J.A. (1980) Head injury. *Nursing Times, 76*:14, 591.

ENGLAND, F.E.C. (1979) Detection of non-accidental injury. *Nursing Times, 75*:43, 1858.

HAYWARD, R. (1980) *Management of Acute Head Injuries*. Oxford: Blackwell Scientific.

JENNET, W.B. (1983) Medical aspects of head injury. *Medicine, 1*:30, 1415.

JENNET, W.B. & TEASDALE, G.M. (1982) *Management of Head Injuries*. Contemporary Neurological Series. Philadelphia: F.A. Davis.

MISIK, I. (1981) About using restraints with restraint. *Nursing (US) 11*:8, 50.

MURDOCH, A.E. (1976) Titanium cranioplasty in the repair of skull defects. *Nursing Times, 72*:37, 1426.

MURDOCH, A.E. (1980) A patient with a depressed fracture of the skull. *Nursing Times, 76*:22, 972.

NIKAS, D.L. (ed.) (1982) *The Critically Ill Neurosurgical Patient*, p. 89. Edinburgh: Churchill Livingstone.

STEVENS, M.M. (1982) Post-concussion syndrome. *Journal of Neurosurgical Nursing, 14*:5, 239.

TEASDALE, G.M. (1975) Acute impairment of brain function-1. Assessing conscious level. *Nursing Times, 71*:24, 914.

TEASDALE, G.M., GALBRAITH, S.L. & CLARKE, K.Y. (1975) Acute impairment of brain function-2. Observation and record chart. *Nursing Times, 71*:25, 972.

YOUNG, J.A. (1981) Head injuries. Advances in care during the last decade. *Nursing Times, 77*:18, 766.

ZEGEER, L.J. (1982) Nursing care of the patient with brain oedema. *Journal of Neurosurgical Nursing, 14*:5, 268.

USEFUL ADDRESS

Headway
National Head Injuries Association
17–21 Clumber Avenue
Sherwood Rise
Nottingham NG5 1AG

6 Care of the unconscious patient

Caring for the unconscious patient can be both extremely frustrating and immensely rewarding for the nurse. A problem-solving approach is the most effective, and to achieve this an assessment is made of the patient's needs, from which a care plan is created. The nurse delivers the care to the patient and then evaluates the effectiveness of her action. The care plan can be altered in the light of new developments in the patient's condition or ineffectual nursing care.

Maintenance of a clear airway

Maintenance of a clear airway is the most important consideration at all times (Fig. 6.1). To achieve this, correct positioning of the

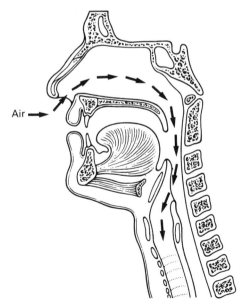

Air →

Fig. 6.1. *Natural airway.*

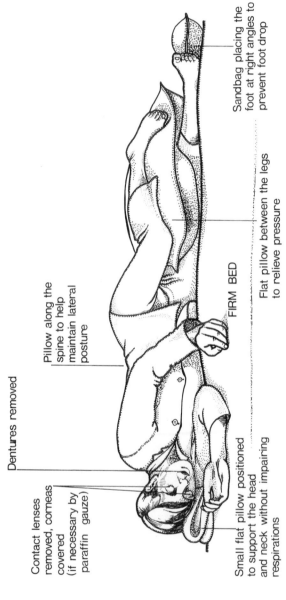

Dentures removed

Pillow along the spine to help maintain lateral posture

Contact lenses removed, corneas covered (if necessary by paraffin gauze)

Small flat pillow positioned to support the head and neck without impairing respirations

FIRM BED

Flat pillow between the legs to relieve pressure

Sandbag placing the foot at right angles to prevent foot drop

Fig. 6.2. *Position of the unconscious patient.*

patient is essential (Fig. 6.2). He should be nursed on his side so that secretions can trickle out of the side of his mouth. The angle of the jaw should be supported to prevent obstruction by the tongue. The patient is placed on his back only if it is absolutely necessary, e.g. for the purpose of intubation, and when in this position is never left unattended. The nurse must watch carefully for signs of inadequate respiration after each repositioning and, if in doubt, seek advice. The patient's head should be suitably supported to avoid suffocation and neck strain.

If his airway is partially blocked, the patient's breathing is often noisy, and cyanosis may be apparent. The reduced oxygen intake leads to cerebral anoxia and an increased carbon dioxide level in the blood, which in turn causes dilatation of the cerebral arteries, thereby adding to existing bleeding or swelling. The patient increases his effort to obtain oxygen and may cough to try to overcome the obstruction. This action raises the venous pressure. The administration of oxygen will help reduce the possibility of cerebral oedema. The monitoring of arterial blood gases is important to ensure that the patient's oxygen and carbon dioxide levels are maintained within normal limits, i.e. pH 7.42; P_{CO_2}, 33–43 mmHg; P_{O_2}, 91–100 mmHg. The most common cause of neurological deterioration is hypoxia.

The usual agents which can endanger the patient's breathing are the tongue, blood, mucus, vomit and dentures. As a safety precaution, the nurse should remove and label the patient's dentures. The insertion of a gastric tube to empty the stomach is advisable in patients who are particularly likely to vomit, e.g. those intoxicated with alcohol.

Blood, mucus and vomit are cleared from the airway by using suction apparatus. Suction should be available and in working order in the admission area and wherever the patient is transferred. The nurse must also ensure that a portable suction machine accompanies the patient while he is being moved.

Disposable plastic airways and intubation equipment should be easily accessible. Before inserting an airway, check that it is the correct size. The presence of an artificial airway does not guarantee an adequate air intake, and the nurse must remain constantly alert to the possibility of obstruction. The air inlet is small and can become blocked with mucus and debris, thereby hindering rather than aiding respiration.

In patients with a compromised cough reflex, endotracheal intubation may be indicated. Most centres advocate the use of soft seal cuffed endotracheal tubes, which reduce the incidence of tracheal ischaemia. Intubated patients need to have an Ambu resuscitation bag, with a swivel connector attached, kept at the bedside. The nurse should be aware of the location of the ward's emergency equipment.

Tracheostomy may be indicated in patients who remain unconscious over a prolonged period of time and cannot maintain an adequate respiratory status. Soft seal cuffed disposable tubes are usually used initially, and these require to be changed every third day. The stoma needs to be kept scrupulously clean, swabbed with an appropriate antiseptic solution, and a dry dressing applied. Tracheal dilators and two spare tracheostomy tubes, one the same size and one a size smaller than the patient's, are kept at the bedside for use in case of accidental dislodgement. If the patient requires a tracheostomy on a more permanent basis, then one of the three-part metal type may be used. This consists of an outer and inner tube with an introducer, the inner tube being removable for easy cleaning.

Observations

Accurate neurological observations are performed to ascertain the patient's level of consciousness and any subsequent improvement or deterioration. A standardised scale is recommended, and a suitable one is the Glasgow Coma Scale (see Chapter 2). A proper coma scale helps to eliminate any confusing or vague terms such as 'stupor' or 'semi-comatose'.

Recording of routine vital signs is indicated and should be performed, along with the neurological observations, every 2 hours.

Oral hygiene

Careful oral hygiene is important in all unconscious patients, and the mouth should be cleaned 2-hourly or more frequently as the need dictates. The mouth should also be checked for any breakdown in the mucosal lining, parotitis or halitosis. The use of a deodorant mouth spray may be indicated.

Eye care

Swabbing of the eyes with normal saline solution to remove debris and discharge should be performed every 2 hours, or more frequently when peri-orbital oedema is present. Some unconscious patients have their eyes open or only partially closed, which leaves the corneas unprotected, in which case artificial teardrops should be instilled and the eyelids taped down. Any signs of infection or damage should be reported so that effective treatment can be initiated.

Feeding

Maintaining adequate nourishment in an unconscious patient is a high priority. A method of feeding should be established within 48 hours of the onset of coma using one of two methods: gastric tube feeding, or parenteral nutrition. Tube feeding is the simpler and most preferred method. The patient should have a nasogastric tube passed and its position checked. It is important to note that patients with basal skull fractures, a history of cerebrospinal rhinorrhoea or nasal injuries should have their gastric tube passed orally. When in doubt, use the oral route.

A minimum intake of 2500 calories is recommended for an average adult; however, the advice of the dietician should be sought in order to establish a suitable feeding regime for each individual. There are many proprietary brands of liquid feed available, and the dietician can best advise which is the most suitable for each patient's needs. A check should be made to see that the patient is absorbing the feed.

The continuous drip feeding method is now advocated as a more natural method rather than giving bolus feeds every 3 hours. Medications can also be given via the gastric tube, obviating the need for repeated injections.

When tube feeding is unsuccessful or contraindicated, the placement of a central line and the administration of i.v. nutrition is indicated. Patients on parenteral nutrition require close observation and should ideally be nursed in an intensive care setting or high dependency unit.

A fairly new method of feeding patients via a peripheral i.v. line has been devised with the advent of Perifusin, an amino acid and electrolyte solution.

Care of the bladder

Catheterisation almost always becomes necessary in unconscious patients. It avoids retention of urine (a common cause of restlessness) and incontinence (a precipitating factor in pressure sores) and allows an accurate check on diuresis. Meticulous 4-hourly catheter care should be performed. The catheter should be taped to the patient's thigh to avoid urethral traction, and the catheter drainage tube attached to the bed to allow for proper drainage.

Care of the bowels

Inactivity and lack of roughage in the diet cause sluggish intestinal movements which often result in constipation. If the patient requires bowel stimulation, Normacol or Senokot granules can be mixed with paraffin emulsion, and gently injected down the gastric tube and flushed with water. Daily aperients and twice-weekly suppositories usually effect two adequate motions, although an enema may occasionally be necessary. Any signs of diarrhoea or constipation should be noted; either may be due to impaction of faeces, inappropriate aperients, or dietary indiscretions. Some patients seem unable to tolerate a full feeding regime for an indefinite period. A sudden bout of diarrhoea can usually be halted by giving the patient water only for 24 hours.

Care of the skin

The patient should be bedbathed once or twice daily as needed. The skin should be inspected at each 2-hourly positional change, particularly over the bony prominences. Any reddened areas should be noted, and measures initiated to regenerate that compromised area of skin. The application of a lubricating lotion will help to combat dry skin.

It may prove useful to predict the unconscious patient's pressure area risk potential with the use of a scoring system such as the Norton scale. With this scale, the patient scores points for each compromise that may add to his potential for pressure sores, and from this the nurse can be alerted as to the degree of risk the patient may be at.

Male patients should be shaved each day.

Care of the hair and nails

The patient's hair should be washed, dried and combed regularly. Nails should be kept clean and short; this is especially important in those patients who clench their fists tightly, lest their nails should dig into the palm of the hand.

Care of the musculoskeletal system

In order to aid rehabilitation, the patient will require to be positioned carefully in bed if complications such as contractures and loss of muscle tone are to be avoided. The patient should have passive range of movement exercises performed every 4 hours as well as good positioning, with any paralysed limbs supported.

Protection of the patient from injury

The mechanism that normally helps people protect themselves from injury does not function in the unconscious patient, thus the nurse must be extra attentive to the needs of this vulnerable group. If the patient suffers a grand mal epileptic seizure, objects that he might strike as his limbs convulse should be removed.

If the patient is being transferred from one area to another, the nurse must ensure that his limbs are not dangling off the trolley and knocking against passing objects. A trolley with side rails will prevent the patient from falling off.

When the unconscious patient is in bed, he is at least risk to injury, provided conscientious care of the skin is maintained. The restless unconscious patient may rub his skin sore, and regular pressure area care is just as important as in the immobile unconscious patient. If the patient is thrashing about the bed, more violent injury may be inflicted, and at this stage padded cot sides and restraints are considered. Regular turning relieves pressure and prevents hypostatic pneumonia.

Care of intravenous infusions

Electrolyte and fluid imbalances can occur easily in the unconscious patient, and so the placement of an i.v. cannula and the infusion of appropriate fluids become necessary. The patient will require regular

monitoring of serum electrolytes and an i.v. fluid regime prescribed according to each set of results. The nurse is responsible for
ensuring that the proper fluids are given at the correct rate. The i.v.
site should be inspected for any signs of inflammation, which should
be documented and reported.

Prevention of infection

As unconscious patients have a lowered resistance to infection, it is
important that the nurse washes her hands before and after performing any procedure for the patient. An aseptic technique should
be adopted when performing procedures such as suctioning the
patient or attending to catheter care.

Control of pain

Unconscious patients can feel pain just the same as anyone else, but
cannot complain or indicate where the pain is. The observant nurse
should be able to tell when the patient is in pain, e.g. he may become
very restless. Analgesia should be prescribed and given.

Avoidance of sensory deprivation

A controlled amount of useful sensory input is vital in the care of the
unconscious patient if the all too common syndrome of sensory
deprivation is to be avoided. The importance of touch cannot be
underestimated. The patient will receive a lot of tactile stimulation
during his physical care, and relatives should be encouraged to hold
the patient's hand.

Auditory stimulation is also important, and this can take the form
of radio, television and the playing of a tape recording of familiar
family voices. The relatives should be encouraged to talk about
familiar everyday topics in order to establish reality and a perspective on time for the patient. However, it is necessary to restrict the
amount of stimulation carefully. It should be borne in mind that if
music is used as a source of stimulation, it should be appropriate to
the patient's age group and taste rather than those of the nurses.

Having the television on 12 hours each day does not constitute
realistic stimulation, and thus frequent rest periods should be incor-

porated in the care plan. It is also unnecessary to shout at the patient or to speak to him in baby talk.

The patient's relatives

Little is known about the states of unconsciousness, and to the involved relative it is not only bewildering, but frightening to see the patient in such a condition. How long will he be unconscious and will he be mentally normal on recovery? These two questions are invariably asked, and equally often cannot be answered. This uncertainty causes further concern to the relatives. The doctor will err on the side of caution when discussing the patient's condition, and it is advisable for relatives to live from day to day rather than for the distant future.

The next of kin will ask if his visits to the unconscious patient are worthwhile, as the patient just lies there, apparently totally out of touch with the world. This question may be prompted by feelings of inadequacy, but the relative can contribute to the patient's care by talking to him. One possible danger of nursing an unconscious patient over a long period of time is that he will be pushed into a corner and kept apart from the rest of the patients.

Although the patient is probably unaware of his detached position, his relatives will not be, and they must never be allowed to feel that the patient is a discarded failure.

FURTHER READING

JONES, D.C. (1975) *Food for Thought.* Series 2, RCN Research Project. London: Royal College of Nursing.

MAUS CLUM, N. (1982) Bringing the unconscious patient back safely. *Nursing (US), 12*:8, 34.

MYCO, F. & McGILLOWAY, F.A. (1980) Care of the unconscious patient, a complementary perspective. *Journal of Advanced Nursing, 5*, 273.

PEMBERTON, L. (1979) Nursing an unconscious patient. *Nursing Mirror, 149*:11, 41.

7 Epilepsy

Epilepsy is one of the most devastating conditions known. It carries many serious implications for the sufferer which involve every aspect of his life. A large number of epileptics cope very well as a result of the understanding and intelligent interest of their families, friends and employers. Unfortunately, widespread ignorance persists with the population at large, who regard epilepsy as something they do not wish to know about. Anyone is capable of having a seizure if the correct conditions exist; however, in epileptics the seizure occurs as a result of a stimulus too small to have an effect on the population at large. This is called the seizure or convulsive threshold. Seizures were first defined in 1870 by John Hughlings Jackson as, 'an occasional excessive and disorderly discharge of nerve tissue', a definition which can still be applied today.

CAUSES

Two broad categories of causes can be identified.

1. Idiopathic (asymptomatic) epilepsy, where there are no structural abnormalities identified and the cause remains unknown.
2. Acquired (symptomatic) epilepsy, where an identifiable lesion is present and may be due to:
   a. head injury;
   b. birth injury or deformities;
   c. systemic cause, e.g. severe infections;
   d. tumours;
   e. local damage, e.g. meningitis or cerebral thrombosis;
   f. metabolic disturbances, e.g. hypoglycaemia;
   g. anoxia;
   h. trigger mechanisms, e.g. flashing lights (reflex epilepsy);
   i. ingestions of toxins, e.g. as in chronic alcoholism.

CLASSIFICATION

Partial seizure disorders

Focal seizures

The term focal epilepsy is used to describe attacks which start in one part of the body and are either limited to this area or may progress to a major convulsion. Such attacks indicate a localised cerebral lesion, the site of which can be diagnosed by the nature of a fit, which may be motor, sensory, auditory or visual. If an attack does spread, it is termed a Jacksonian fit, and one of the commonest encountered is where a motor cortex lesion gives rise to a convulsion that often starts in the corner of the mouth, or at the thumb and index finger, progresses down that side of the body and may involve the opposite limbs in a generalised fit with loss of consciousness. The length of the attack is usually 2–3 minutes, but it may last up to an hour, and can be followed by a weakness of the convulsed part. This temporary state is called Todd's paralysis.

Temporal lobe epilepsy

Lesions located within the temporal lobe may give rise to temporal lobe epilepsy. The aura (the first manifestation of a seizure) may either be the only feature, or the attack may progress to a generalised seizure. The aura may consist of a strange abdominal sensation associated with a *déjà-vu* phenomenon, i.e. where the patient feels that he recognises his present situation because he has lived through it before. At the onset of the seizure, there may be an alteration or loss of consciousness.

Following a seizure, a patient may exhibit automatic behaviour: he repeats a seemingly purposeless action vigorously, e.g. clapping his hands. Aggressive repetitive actions may also be a feature, and are termed postepileptic automatism. The patient is amnesic of such acts when he regains consciousness.

Generalised seizure disorders

Grand mal seizures

These can be subdivided into several distinct stages.

The aura. A premonitory sensation, which may consist of light or a curious epigastric sensation, this occurs in about half of those people with grand mal seizures.

The tonic phase. The patient often cries out as he loses consciousness. He falls to the ground and becomes stiff, with rigid limbs. The respiratory muscles are also affected causing cyanosis. This phase will last 25–45 seconds.

The clonic phase. This is a phase in which the rigidity subsides to be replaced by rhythmic jerks which gradually become less frequent. There may be biting of the tongue, urinary and faecal incontinence, and frothing at the mouth. This stage may last for 1–2 minutes and is followed by coma.

Coma. The patient will lapse into an unconscious state with flaccid limbs, lasting up to 2 hours. Thoroughly exhausted from his exertions, the patient will sleep soundly and when awakened he may be very drowsy, confused or amnesic and complain of headache. Many patients will depart from this well-recognised pattern, and several variations may be observed.

Petit mal seizures

Petit mal epilepsy is usually confined to childhood years and terminates, for most sufferers, during their teenage years. It is characterised by a momentary alteration of consciousness, so that the patient may pause in conversation and/or take on a vacant look. The entire episode passes over in seconds, and indeed many observers may not be aware that the patient has just had a seizure. There are rarely any after-effects or loss of consciousness.

Myoclonic seizures

The patient sustains a sudden short shock-like jerk of a limb or of his body. There is usually no detectable loss of consciousness. Myoclonus is sometimes included with the petit mal group of seizures.

Akinetic seizures

These consist of a sudden loss of movement with no loss of consciousness.

Infantile convulsions

The vast majority of convulsions in children are temperature related rather than epileptogenic. In 'salaam' fits, the child flexes his trunk, with extension of both arms and drawing-up of the legs.

Status epilepticus

One seizure, usually of the grand mal type, follows on rapidly from another without the patient recovering consciousness. The patient may suffer brain damage as a result of the intermittent hypoxia caused by repeated respiratory obstruction.

The most common cause of status epilepticus is withdrawal of anti-epileptic medication in a chronic sufferer.

DIAGNOSIS

A diagnosis of epilepsy must only be made following careful consideration of the history and a thorough examination. A reliable eye-witness account from a reliable observer remains one of the best ways of confirming that a seizure has occurred.

Various points need to be noted.

Was there an aura?
Did the patient lose consciousness?
In which part of the body did the seizure start and how did it proceed?
What type of movement was observed?
Were there any changes in pupillary size or reaction?
Was there any incontinence?
Was any injury sustained?
What was the duration of the attack?
Did the patient complain of any after-effects?

A full neurological and physical examination should be performed in order to eliminate any underlying pathology which may be causing the seizures (and so require further investigation) and to establish any possible differential diagnosis, e.g. syncope. An electroencephalogram (EEG) merely classifies rather than diagnoses the type of epilepsy. Known abnormal wave patterns are produced in certain types of epilepsy.

The results of the EEG must be kept in perspective with the rest of the history and assessment. A small percentage of the population will display abnormal EEG patterns but clinically are fit and well, while 10% of those people with well-documented seizures will display a normal EEG.

When the cause of the seizures is due to an underlying lesion, this needs to be investigated using any of the full range of diagnostic procedures previously mentioned in Chapter 3.

TREATMENT

The aim of treatment is to prevent seizures so that the patient can lead as normal a life as possible. The treatment plan is modified to suit each patient's individual needs, and may be composed of one or more of the following:

- a. drug therapy;
- b. surgical treatment;
- c. rehabilitation.

Drug therapy

The aim is to reduce the excitability of the nerve cells, and this can be achieved with the use of one or more of the anticonvulsants listed in Table 7.1. Sometimes a combination of two drugs may be used, which enables the patient to reduce the dosage of a medication (which may have unacceptable side-effects) while retaining good seizure control. Side-effects and signs of toxicity must be watched for during routine screening sessions, which will also include the monitoring of serum drug levels. Potentially dangerous drug interactions must be avoided, e.g. phenytoin sodium will potentiate the action of many antihypertensive agents and inhibit the action of steroids. Emphasis must be placed on taking the medication regularly, as one of the most common causes of seizure activity is the withdrawal of anticonvulsant therapy. Any changes in the drug regime must be gradual and made only under medical supervision.

Table 7.1 *Anticonvulsants used in the treatment of epilepsy.*

Drug	Average adult daily dose	Use	Side-effects	Remarks
Phenytoin sodium (Epanutin)	100–400 mg	Grand mal and psychomotor epilepsy	Dizziness, nausea, skin reactions, gingival hyperplasia, ataxia, nystagmus	
Phenobarbitone (Luminal)	60–400 mg	Grand mal and all partial seizures	Drowsiness, dizziness, ataxia, physical dependence	
Diazepam (Valium)	4–40 mg	Status epilepticus (5–10 mg i.v.)	Fatigue, drowsiness, ataxia	Causes respiratory depression
Paraldehyde	5–10 ml	Status epilepticus	Local irritations at site of injection	Very safe anticonvulsant
Chlormethiazole (Heminevrin)	40–100 ml i.v. 0·8% sol	Status epilepticus	May cause respiratory depression	Slow i.v.
Carbamezapine (Tegretol)	200–1200 mg	Grand mal and temporal lobe epilepsy	Dizziness, rash, psychotic behaviour	
Clonazepam (Rivitrol)	20 mg	Myoclonic seizures and petit mal	Rash, thrombocytopenia, ataxia, hyper-salivation	
Ethosuximide (Zarontin)	0·5–2·0 g	Petit mal	Drowsiness and gastric upset	May aggravate grand mal
Primidone (Mysoline)	0·5–2·0 g	Grand mal and psychomotor epilepsy	Well tolerated	
Sodium valporate (Epilim)	600 mg increasing by 200 mg daily at 3-day intervals to a maximum of 2·6 g	Grand mal and petit mal	Gastric upset	
Sulthiame (Ospolot)	200 mg increasing to 600 mg	Temporal lobe epilepsy	Paraesthesia of face, gastric disturbances, headache	

Surgical treatment

Surgical treatment is indicated in those cases with an identifiable lesion, e.g. a tumour. Patients with temporal lobe epilepsy may be improved by the removal of part of the non-dominant temporal lobe, if this is the site of the epileptogenic focus.

For the vast majority of epileptic patients, surgery plays no part in their treatment.

Rehabilitation

An individualised and well-organised teaching plan is necessary to make the patient's discharge and subsequent life as unobtrusive as possible. Discharge planning starts on the day the patient is admitted. The attitude of the nurse and, to a lesser extent, the doctor, will help to dispel the prevailing prejudices which exist in regard to epilepsy.

The patient's family should be involved in the teaching programme, and the following points need to be covered.

Drugs

These must be taken on a regular basis, even though the patient may have a prolonged seizure-free period. A schedule which will remind the patient when to take his medication may be useful. The patient must be reminded of the need to attend the out-patient clinic regularly for routine screening. Some patients may be asked to keep a written record of when their seizures occur in relation to when they take their medication. At the clinic, serum drug levels will be monitored and drug regimes altered to obtain the optimum benefit for the patient. The patient needs to be warned of the potential side-effects of his drugs and signs and symptoms of toxicity.

Trigger mechanisms

Certain situations may trigger off seizure activity for some patients, and they need to be warned of this. Such trigger mechanisms may include: inadequate serum drug levels; illness; lack of sleep; emotional stress; hormonal changes such as occur with menstruation; poor nutrition; or electrolyte imbalance.

Social rehabilitation

Complete abstention from alcohol will be required as alcohol inhibits the action of many anticonvulsants and, accordingly, alcohol will cause the patient's susceptibility to a seizure to increase dramatically. Women should consult with their doctors before considering pregnancy, so that they can be advised of the risks involved and how best to minimise them. Epileptics should be encouraged to engage in their normal physical activities; however, dangerous sports such as mountain climbing should be avoided.

Precautions

If a few simple precautions are taken, then the epileptic's life at home will be a lot less traumatic. Having a shower rather than a bath is safer for the patient, but when this is not possible, bathing with supervision or at least with the bathroom door open and someone nearby to help if necessary is advisable. Informing workmates of what to do should the epileptic have a seizure will enlighten their attitude, and the episode will not be so frightening for them.

The patient should always carry an identification card detailing name, address, information telling passers-by what to do should the patient sustain a seizure, and a contact telephone number. A useful alternative is the Medic-Alert jewellery.

Driving restrictions

The patient will need to be informed of driving restrictions. An epileptic can only get a licence if:

  a. he is free of seizures for three years, while awake;
  b. has suffered seizures while asleep only;
  c. is not likely to be a danger to the public while driving.

The driving licence needs to be renewed annually.

Employment

This can pose considerable problems for the patient. If his job involved driving or working with moving machinery, this would present as a serious danger. For many patients, the available options are unacceptable: if they attend an interview for a job, they are frequently turned down because of their epilepsy; on the other hand, if they do not reveal their problem, then they run the risk of having a seizure at work and being dismissed for withholding the information at the interview.

Related nursing skills

When a known epileptic or someone who is thought to have

epilepsy is admitted to hospital, certain routine precautions must be taken to protect the patient from possible injury. These precautions should, where possible, he discussed with the patient in order that he understands why they are necessary.

Padded bedrails should be used and maintained in the up position whilst the patient is asleep and during the night. The patient should be kept under unobtrusive observation while showering, and it is safer if he avoids taking baths. Smoking should not be permitted in bed. The patient's temperature should never be taken orally or rectally. A tongue depressor, oral airway, oxygen and suction should be located nearby.

Nursing action during a seizure

Should a patient sustain a seizure, the nurse must remain calm and confident. Several immediate needs must be attended to, including the following.

1. Maintain a clear airway; roll the patient onto his side, loosen tight clothing and establish the location of oxygen and suction. Some sources advocate placing a gag between the patient's teeth in order to prevent tongue biting, however, in practice, this is rarely possible. It is improbable that a nurse would be present at the moment a seizure starts and is more likely to arrive on the scene a few seconds later, by which time the patient has entered the clonic phase, making it impossible and unwise to force a gag into place.
2. Summon help.
3. Prevent the patient from injuring himself; place a pillow under his head and use gentle restraint only.
4. Record on a seizure chart the duration, severity and a description of the seizure.
5. Constant reassurance should be given to the patient throughout the seizure: speak to the patient in a quiet, relaxed manner.
6. Ensure privacy for the patient and allay onlookers.
7. When prescribed, the appropriate anticonvulsant should be administered. Any i.v. sites will need to be protected during the seizure lest the cannula is accidentally dislodged.

If the seizures continue unabated, then status epilepticus has developed and further intervention is required.

1. Maintenance of a clear airway remains a high priority. While the patient fits continually, this becomes more difficult to achieve and therefore oxygen and suction must be readily available and used. The patient should not be left unattended.
2. A written record is kept of the number and type of seizures.
3. Administration of further anticonvulsants will be required (see Table 7.1), and appropriate medication includes diazepam (Valium), paraldehyde, or chlormethiazole (Hemineverin).
4. If these measures do not work, the use of an anaesthetic agent such as thiopentone (Pentothal) may be considered. This is given intravenously and the patient requires intubation and ventilatory support.
5. With so much energy being expended as a result of increased muscle activity, the temperature often rises very quickly. As this will make increased demands on the patient's oxygen uptake, it is important that measures are taken to reduce the pyrexia. These measures can include fanning, tepid sponging, or the use of antipyretic medication.
6. Hydration is maintained with intravenous fluids. Careful fixation of the cannula is necessary so that it is not dislodged by the repeated convulsing.

FURTHER READING

DRAPER, I.T. (1980) *Lecture Notes on Neurology*, 5th edn., p. 83. Oxford: Blackwell Scientific.

FENWICK, P., PERKINS, H. & BRETT, E.M. (1978) Epilepsy Symposium (part II). *Nursing Mirror, 147*:5, 13.

HOPKINS, A. (1981) *Epilepsy — the facts*. London: Oxford University Press.

KOSHY, K.T. (1975) A comprehensive look at epilepsy. *Nursing Times, 71*:26, 1013.

LAIDLAW, M.V. & LAIDLAW, J. (1980) *Epilepsy Explained — a Patient Handbook*. Edinburgh: Churchill Livingstone.

LINDSAY, M. (1982) Living with epilepsy-1. *Nursing Times, 78*:26, 1115.

LINDSAY, M. (1982) Epilepsy-2. People with epilepsy in the job market. *Nursing Times, 78*:27, 1155.

NORMAN, S.E., BROWNE, T.R. & TUCKER, C.A. (1981) Seizure disorders. *American Journal of Nursing, 81*:5, 983.

OXLEY, J., BETTS, T. & NAYLOR, P. (1981) Epilepsy — clinical forum 12. *Nursing Mirror, 153*: 24.

REYNOLDS, E.H., KELLY, J. & SHORVON, S.D. (1978) Epilepsy Symposium (part I). *Nursing Mirror, 147*:4.

ROBINSON, N. (1982) Epidemiology of epilepsy. *Nursing Times. 78*:41, 1717.

TREKAS, J. (1982) Managing epilepsy: don't forget the patient. *Nursing (US)*, *12*:10, 63.

USEFUL ADDRESSES

British Epilepsy Association
Crowthorne House
New Wokingham Road
Wokingham
Berkshire RG11 3AY

Medic-Alert Foundation
9 Hanover Street
London WIR 9HF

8   Infections

Inflammation of the nervous system is usually due to infection, which may be acute or chronic. The causative organisms are bacteria, viruses and fungi. The clinical features, and therefore the related nursing skills, depend on the site and duration of the infection.

The infections are summarised as follows:

acute meningitis
chronic meningitis
infections involving the nervous tissue
neurosyphilis
peripheral neuritis

ACUTE MENINGITIS

Acute bacterial (pyogenic) meningitis, once a common and frequently fatal disease, is now largely avoided because infections located elsewhere in the body, to which the disease is often secondary, have been treated earlier and more effectively since the introduction of antibiotics. Any pathogenic organism can cause this disease once the subarachnoid space is penetrated, but the commonest are the meningococcus, which may give rise to epidemics, the pneumococcus, *Haemophilus influenzae* (only in infants) and *Escherichia coli* (confined to neonates). A rash may be apparent.

Many viral infections are associated with a mild meningitis, e.g. mumps, measles, glandular fever. Those that mainly affect the meninges mostly belong to the enterovirus group, which invade the body from the alimentary tract, e.g. the coxsackie viruses and the poliomyelitis virus.

The infective agent usually gains access to the nervous system via the bloodstream, although some bacteria spread from an adjacent septic source such as a nasal sinus infection, and some viruses travel along nerves, e.g. herpes virus.

Clinical features

In acute meningitis, the patient has a raised temperature, is flushed, and complains of a severe headache associated with photophobia. He tries to relax and relieve tension by adopting a position of lying curled up with his legs flexed, his head extended and neck rigid. Attempts to flex the neck cause muscular spasm and consequent neck stiffness. Similarly, if the knee and hip are flexed at right angles, straightening the knee causes severe pain and spasm of the hamstrings (Kernig's sign). Both tests are used to confirm meningism (Figs. 8.1 and 8.2). Hyperextension of the back and neck (opisthotonus) is characteristic in infants, and convulsions are common. If the patient is severely infected, he will become drowsy, irritable and delirious and will eventually lapse into coma if the disease continues unchecked.

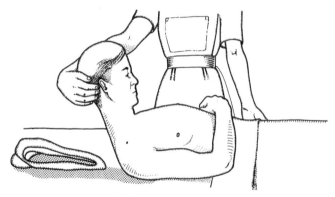

Fig. 8.1. *Test for meningism.*

Diagnosis

Patients with suspected meningitis, and all very ill infants, should have a lumbar puncture and an examination of the cerebrospinal fluid to confirm or disprove the diagnosis. One or two nurses (depending on the patient's co-operation) will be needed to assist the doctor in this procedure.

In pyogenic meningitis, the cerebrospinal fluid is turbid, and analysis shows polymorphs (more than 500/mm^3), a raised protein level (0.5–1.0 g/l) and reduced sugar content (less than 2.5 mmol/l).

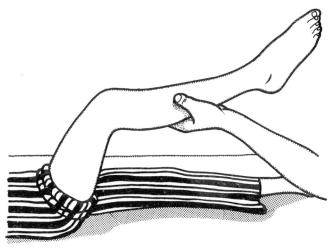

Fig. 8.2. *Test for Kernig's sign.*

The presence and identity of the causative organism are established.

In viral (aseptic) meningitis, the cerebrospinal fluid is clear or slightly cloudy, and analysis shows lymphocytes (up to 200/mm³) and a raised protein level. The sugar content is normal and no organisms are seen, but sometimes viruses can be cultured.

Treatment of bacterial meningitis

Intrathecal or intravenous antibiotic therapy should be commenced as soon as the diagnosis has been made and before the cerebrospinal fluid is cultured. Large doses of penicillin (Crystapen) 12–18 g daily are often given, and ampicillin (Penbritin), sulphadiazine (Sulphadimidine), cephaloridine (Ceporin) or occasionally chloramphenicol (Chloromycetin) may be used once the causative organism is identified. Intravenous injections of antibiotics are more comfortable for the patient and produce a more rapid effect. Once the acute phase has passed, therapy is maintained with intramuscular injections.

Intrathecal penicillin is specially prepared by the pharmacist in a small quantity (20 000 i.u.) and with no preservative so that damage to the spinal cord is avoided. Daily lumbar puncture and cerebrospinal fluid analysis enable the doctor to inject intrathecal penicillin as required, assess the patient's response to the treatment, and plan future antibiotic therapy. Side-effects from these drugs may occur. In particular, chloramphenicol can lead to blood dyscrasia.

When meningitis is secondary to an adjacent focus of infection, such as an ear abscess or sinusitis, the appropriate surgical treatment is required. On rare occasions, the infection produces a fistula through which cerebrospinal fluid leaks, and any drainage of clear fluid from the ear or nose should be noted. The defect in the dura may seal itself but should otherwise be repaired in 7–10 days to reduce the risk of re-infection.

Related nursing skills

The patient should be nursed in a darkened side room because of his photophobia, and given frequent analgesics, e.g. codeine phosphate 30–60 mg, to control headache. When the temperature is raised, measures must be taken to reduce it, i.e. tepid sponging, cool fanning and/or aspirin suppositories. The patient, who will be sweating profusely, must receive a fluid intake of at least 2500 ml daily, and the oral administration of this amount to a drowsy and irritable patient may be difficult. Whether or not feeding via a nasogastric tube or i.v. infusion becomes necessary, the patient must be given regular oral hygiene. Careful neurological observations will detect any change in the patient's condition and, when he is in coma, the nursing care explained in Chapter 6 is applicable.

In addition to the above measures, patients with bacterial meningitis must be barrier nursed because they are infectious. Strictly maintained precautions to prevent the disease spreading are instituted and, although it is preferable to nurse the patient in a single room, a corner of the ward screened off near the sluice is a satisfactory alternative. Whichever area is used, it should have a 'Barrier Nursing' notice strategically placed to prevent unsuspecting persons entering unprotected. Anyone who visits the patient must wear a mask and a gown, not only for their own safety, but to prevent them from being carriers of the bacteria. A supply of disposable masks is kept outside the infected area. On discarding the mask into a disposable bag, only the taping should be touched. All waste paper, food and mouth swabs are wrapped in a strong disposable bag and then dropped into a thick paper sack at the entrance to the contaminated area. This is carefully fastened with staples and marked 'Infected: for Burning'.

The side of the gown which comes into contact with the patient is 'dirty' and that next to the wearer 'clean', and these must not be mixed up. The gown is kept on a coathanger in the infected area with the dirty side outwards and, if two are used, they are hung facing each other. The coathanger, which is also kept clean, facilitates the donning of the gown without contaminating it. The gowns are changed every 24 hours and also if they become wet. After touching the patient or the gown, the hands must be thoroughly washed and dried. Any articles inside the room must not be removed without the appropriate measures to disinfect them, and therefore the patient's notes and x-rays remain outside. All linen is placed in a plastic bag and, at the entrance to the isolated area, dropped carefully into an uncontaminated bag, securely tied and labelled 'Infected linen'.

The contents are soaked in a disinfectant before being laundered and returned to the general linen supply. Feeding utensils and equipment used to collect excreta must be marked with the patient's name and cleaned separately (and extra thoroughly) from the ward's articles.

When the patient is no longer infected, the bedding is autoclaved and the whole area is either washed with disinfectant and aired thoroughly or, if a separate room is used, it may be closed and fumigated.

Complications of bacterial meningitis

Fibrinous adhesions may form in the subarachnoid space, obstructing the flow of cerebrospinal fluid, and leading to hydrocephalus and dementia. The inflammation may damage the cranial nerves, especially the optic and auditory, resulting in blindness and deafness respectively.

Treatment of viral meningitis

Viral meningitis is much less severe than bacterial meningitis and usually resolves spontaneously, with the patient making a complete recovery. Treatment is limited to general nursing care.

CHRONIC MENINGITIS

The signs and symptoms of chronic meningitis evolve over the course of several days or weeks, rather than hours as in acute meningitis. The most important infective agent is the tubercle bacillus, but syphilis, some fungi and infiltration of the meninges by malignant cells, can also cause meningitis.

Tuberculous meningitis

If this condition is not treated, there is a 100% mortality rate. Antituberculous drug therapy reduces this to about 20%, although many of the survivors have serious neurological defects, e.g. deafness, blindness, hydrocephalus or dementia from cerebral adhesions, or paraplegia from spinal cord adhesions.

Tuberculous meningitis occurs most frequently in young children, who present with drowsiness, fits and focal neurological signs. Headaches and intellectual impairment mark the insidious onset in adults, followed by loss of appetite and general malaise. To confirm the diagnosis, a lumbar puncture is performed which reveals an increased cerebrospinal fluid pressure, high protein content and a raised cell count (generally lymphocytes). The sugar level is low and the presence of tubercle bacilli is usually demonstrated. There may be evidence of tuberculous infection elsewhere in the body, and a chest x-ray and examination of the urine for tubercle bacilli should also be performed.

Treatment is with specific antituberculous drugs. Streptomycin is given intramuscularly (0.5 g twice daily). Oral para-aminosalicylic acid (PAS) 12 g/day and isoniazid (INAH) 300 mg/day are usually given in combination. Rifampicin capsules 450 mg/day are also used. Treatment with two or more of the drugs is imperative in order to prevent the development of antibiotic resistance in the tubercle bacillus. The treatment must be continued for at least one year.

Steroid therapy is often used with the aim of reducing the severity of post-inflammatory adhesions, which cause much of the morbidity of this illness.

Prolonged antituberculous drug therapy may produce unwanted side-effects. Streptomycin can damage the eighth cranial nerve, causing permanent deafness or unsteadiness, and is particularly likely to do so if drug excretion is prevented because of impairment in renal function. Para-aminosalicylic acid often causes gastric irritation.

Fungal meningitis

The clinical picture of a patient with fungal meningitis resembles that of tuberculous meningitis. This rare disease is difficult to treat because antifungal agents are very toxic when given systemically.

Malignant meningitis

Malignant meningitis can be found in patients with terminal disseminated carcinoma, usually of the breast or bronchus, but also where no primary tumour is obvious, and in cases of acute leukaemia. Treatment consists of tackling the underlying malignant disease and administering cytotoxic drugs, e.g. methotrexate, systemically and intrathecally.

Syphilitic meningitis

See Neurosyphilis (p. 124).

INFECTIONS INVOLVING THE NERVOUS TISSUE

Bacterial infection of the nervous system is usually localised as an abscess which behaves as a space-occupying lesion.

Acute infective intracranial lesion

Cerebral abscesses

The intact dura is an excellent barrier against foreign bodies entering the brain, and most abscesses are secondary to other body infections. Cerebral infection may be introduced by:

   a.   blood-borne metastasis from a focus of infection elsewhere in the body, e.g. bronchiectasis or infected heart valve, when the abscess may develop in any part of the brain;
   b.   breaching of the dura, e.g. occurring as a result of open head injury or at operation;

c. direct spread from a neighbouring infection, e.g. frontal sinusitis leads to abscess in the frontal lobe, and middle ear infection spreads upwards into the temporal lobe or backwards into the cerebellum.

When bacteria enter the brain, the area in which they settle becomes oedematous and swollen and then liquefies as white blood cells enter to form pus. The brain tries to wall off the abscess with a fibrous capsule which becomes thicker in time. The abscess enlarges and acts as a space-occupying lesion. Focal signs are appropriate to the site: frontal lobe abscesses often cause fits, those in the temporal lobe lead to mild dysphasia, and cerebellar lesions give rise to nystagmus and ataxia.

Death may occur from coning or rupture of the abscess into the ventricular system. The abscess may be located with the use of enhanced CT scanning. Isotope scanning and electroencephalography may also be useful. The cerebrospinal fluid contains lymphocytes and/or polymorphs. Plain x-rays may show a lung abscess or chronic infection in a frontal sinus or the mastoid region.

Treatment. The patient is acutely ill, with a fluctuating conscious level, and although both the cerebral infection and its source demand urgent treatment, the space-occupying lesion takes priority.

A burr hole is made over the abscess and a needle passed into its cavity. The pus is aspirated and samples are sent for bacteriological analysis so that the appropriate massive doses of systemic antibiotics are continued. Penicillin and/or streptomycin may be injected into the cavity. Until the pus dries up, the abscess may be aspirated daily and its size assessed by CT scanning. At a later date, the remaining scar may be excised to reduce the risk of epilepsy. Anticonvulsants are given prophylactically for up to 3 years following supratentorial abscess.

If the abscess is secondary to otitis media or frontal sinusitis, an ear, nose and throat surgeon should drain the infected area.

Very occasionally, infection enters the subdural space and, because there are no barriers, it spreads rapidly over the whole cerebral hemisphere. Focal fits occur and often lead to status epilepticus. A hemiplegia develops as the veins draining the cerebral cortex thrombose. Unless the abscess is drained by multiple burr holes and the subdural space irrigated with solutions containing penicillin, coma and death supervene within 24–48 hours. Systemic antibiotics and anticonvulsants are given. The overall mortality rate is about 40%.

Chronic infective intracranial lesions

Tuberculous lesions

A tuberculoma is a chronic granuloma due to tuberculosis. It usually occurs in a cerebellar hemisphere and is a common intracranial mass in countries where tuberculosis is rife.

Viral encephalitis

The viruses of mumps, measles and glandular fever can all cause a central nervous system infection. The patient has a headache and is confused and drowsy, although these features are usually mild in comparison to the generalised upset to which treatment is primarily directed. Occasionally, the encephalitis is so severe that diagnosis of the systemic illness is obscured. As previously stated, certain viruses, e.g. coxsackie viruses and the poliomyelitis virus, affect the nervous system predominantly, and some produce epidemics of meningoencephalitis. Very rarely, encephalitis may follow a smallpox vaccination.

Related nursing skills. Nursing care of the patient with encephalitis is basically the same as for the patient with meningitis. An intake of at least 2500 ml of fluid must be given by the appropriate method, and regular analgesics administered to ease headache. If the patient becomes unconscious, full nursing care is needed to maintain adequate ventilation of the lungs, a balanced diet, intact skin and correct positioning of the body and limbs, and normal bladder and bowel functions (see Chapter 6).

Hemiplegia and fits may develop, and the nurse must be alert to these possibilities, recording and reporting any such variations in the patient's condition. Anticonvulsant therapy is employed if fits occur. In epidemics of encephalitis it should be assumed that the patient is infectious. Barrier nursing is instituted, with special care being given to the disposal of faeces and the sterilisation of bedpans.

Herpes simplex encephalitis

This encephalitis deserves a special mention as it is the most severe form occurring in the UK. The herpes simplex organism is responsible for cold sores. The development of encephalitis is usually confined to patients who have not been infected previously by the virus. Headaches, behaviour disturbances and hallucinations are the usual presenting features, and these may lead to the patient being admitted to a psychiatric hospital. However, progressive drowsiness and fits soon indicate the presence of a serious organic disease.

The virus attacks the temporal lobes predominantly, often asymmetrically so that hemiplegia, aphasia and focal fits are common. There may be massive swelling of one or both temporal lobes, leading to pressure-cone formation and death from mid-brain compression. In untreated cases, the mortality rate is 70% and the majority of survivors have severe residual neurological deficits. Severe disturbances of memory are almost inevitable because both temporal lobes are damaged.

Treatment. Steroid therapy (dexamethasone) helps to reduce the swelling, and thus mortality. Antiviral agents, e.g. acyclovir (Zovirax), can also be used.

Rabies

The rabies virus, which is usually transmitted by the bite of an infected animal, travels along the nerve tracts to the central nervous system, where it causes an encephalitis which is invariably fatal. The incubation period varies from 9 days up to 12 months, and then the symptoms of malaise, pain and tingling at the site of the wound develop. Within a few days the patient becomes restless and irritable and his voice weakens. Attempts to drink cause spasm of the laryngeal muscles and this leads to the characteristic symptom of fear of water (hydrophobia). Generalised weakness occurs, followed by coma, convulsions and death.

There is no curative treatment once symptoms have developed and prophylaxis is very important.

General preventive measures. The UK is one of the very few countries free of rabies, and to stop the disease being imported, all warm-blooded animals are quarantined for 6 months on arrival. In less fortunate countries where rabies is endemic, stray dogs are caught and destroyed to prevent the spread of the disease.

Treatment. The vigorousness of treatment depends on the severity of the wounds and the state of the animal. If the bites are extensive or the animal is obviously infected, an injection of serum containing antibodies is given (passive immunisation), followed by a 14-day course of intraperitoneal vaccine containing killed virus (active immunisation), with booster doses after a further 10 and 20 days.

When a slight wound is inflicted by an apparently healthy animal, the area is cleaned and the animal caged for 10 days. If the animal cannot be caught, or if it develops signs of rabies during the period of quarantine, a course of vaccine is started immediately.

Related nursing skills. Nursing care is symptomatic. A quiet, darkened room helps to reduce the effect of cerebral irritation, and regular doses of a sedative, e.g. chlorpromazine, are given so that the patient's suffering is lessened. The care of the rabid patient is distressing to all involved, and the feelings of inadequacy extend to the relatives, who will need considerable comfort and support as the disease takes its horrific course.

Encephalitis lethargica

Encephalitis lethargica, which mainly affects the brainstem, was seen in epidemics between 1915 and 1930, but since then has not recurred. Presumed to have been a virus infection, its features were drowsy days and wakeful nights, with ocular palsies and pupillary abnormalities, and in some cases hiccuping occurred. Some of the sufferers later developed an extrapyramidal rigidity, similar to that seen in Parkinson's disease, i.e. post-encephalitic parkinsonism. This complication was permanent and is still encountered in the occasional elderly patient.

Viral myelitis

The commonest viral infection of the spinal cord is anterior poliomyelitis.

Anterior poliomyelitis

Anterior poliomyelitis is so called because it affects the motor cells in the anterior horn of the grey matter in the spinal cord. The causative organism is the enterovirus, which inhabits the intestine. It enters through the mouth and is transmitted in the excreta. Great care has to be taken in the disposal of faeces, which must be soaked for 2 hours in disinfectant. The hands should be washed after defaecation and before preparing meals.

Clinical features. The incubation period is 7 to 21 days, and the infection is usually asymptomatic (i.e. detectable only by antibody changes in the blood), or else develops into a mild illness with sore throat, aching limbs and pyrexia. A small number of patients develop aseptic meningitis (non-paralytic poliomyelitis), and in about 1% paralytic poliomyelitis occurs. Flaccid paralysis is usually preceded by cramp-like pains, muscular spasm and undue sensi-tivity of the skin. Any or all of the motor system may be involved, and weakness may be mild or severe, and slow or very rapid in progression. Paralysis is generally most marked around injection sites, e.g. for triple vaccine or operation wounds. These procedures are avoided during epidemics of poliomyelitis. Involvement of the brainstem nuclei causes cranial nerve palsies, e.g. facial weakness and squints, and respiratory failure. On rare occasions encephalitis may occur.

Diagnosis. The cerebrospinal fluid reveals a high protein content and increased numbers of lymphocytes, and the virus may be cul-tured from a specimen of faeces. An increase in the antibody titre in the blood confirms diagnosis.

Treatment and related nursing skills. The treatment and nursing care of the paralysed conscious patient are described under acute infective polyneuritis, but in addition to these measures, barrier nursing must be instituted for 3 weeks because poliomyelitis is contagious.

The duration of the illness and of the patient's stay in hospital is often long, and he will need every support from his family and the staff caring for him. In particular, the nurses are continuously present and can contribute greatly in keeping his morale high so that he works hard to regain power in his limbs. The occupational therapist instructs him in the use of devices to overcome his disabilities and also provides diversional activities to reduce boredom. Regular visits by relatives are important during long periods of hospitalisation, and many patients appreciate talks with a priest or chaplain. When there are domestic or financial problems, the social worker may be able to help.

Prevention. Immunisation with live, attenuated virus taken orally on a sugar lump is widespread in many countries and has very greatly reduced the world incidence of the disease. The vaccine virus colonises the bowel and prevents the invasion of virulent organisms. During epidemics, public baths and swimming pools are closed to reduce the risk of cross-infection.

Prognosis and long-term after-effects. Of patients with paralytic poliomyelitis, up to 5% of children and 25% of adults die. If the bulbar muscles are involved, the mortality rate is even higher.

Many patients with paralytic poliomyelitis recover completely. About 60% of the power returns in 3 months, with slower improvement continuing for up to 2 years. The muscles which remain paralysed become wasted. Of the less fortunate patients who are permanently disabled, some are wheelchair bound, and a very small number remain completely paralysed and dependent on a respirator.

If a child suffers paralysis of the muscles of one leg, this limb grows less than the other so that on standing the pelvis becomes tilted and a severe scoliosis results. A shoe raised on the affected side will counteract this, and sometimes the complex treatment of halting growth of the normal limb is considered.

The skin of a severely paralysed limb may become atrophic, cold, blue and painful and these symptoms are often reduced by sympathectomy.

In later life, between the ages of 40 and 50 years, some patients complain that weak muscles are becoming weaker and more wasted. The cause of this is not clear.

Herpes zoster (shingles)

A description of the nerves that the herpes zoster virus attacks and the treatment of post-herpetic neuralgia are given in Chapter 19. It is briefly mentioned here as the muscles supplied by the affected nerve root may become paralysed, and occasionally transverse myelitis occurs with loss of function of the spinal cord below the level of the lesion.

NEUROSYPHILIS

Syphilis is caused by a micro-organism, the spirochaete *Treponema pallidum*, and is usually transmitted by sexual intercourse; it is therefore classed as a sexually transmitted disease. Occasionally, infection crosses the placenta and produces congenital syphilis in the infant. Early in the course of infection (4 to 8 weeks after exposure) the meninges and nervous system are involved and there may be signs and symptoms of meningitis. Clinical recovery occurs in all cases, but a small proportion of patients develop complications several years later.

There are three main clinical pictures, but many patients show a mixture of these.

Meningovascular (cerebrospinal) syphilis

Five to ten years after the initial infection, the spirochaete causes inflammation and thickening of the meninges and blood vessels, resulting in thrombosis. These, in turn, give diverse and varying degrees of neurological damage, e.g. fits, hemiplegia or paraplegia.

General paralysis of the insane

General paralysis of the insane is produced by occlusion of many microscopic arteries in the cerebral cortex, leading to atrophy. The clinical features are progressive dementia, fits and spastic quadriparesis. Tremors, emotional lability and delusions are common. Delusions of grandeur (e.g. the patient imagines he is Napoleon) are said to be characteristic of the disease.

Tabes dorsalis

Occurring up to 20 years after the primary infections, tabes dorsalis causes atrophy of the nerve fibres in the sensory tracts of the spinal cord, leading to loss of joint position sense so that the patient walks with an ataxic, stamping gait.

Loss of pain sensation allows injuries to go unheeded, and from relatively minor trauma, ulceration of the feet and swollen disorganised joints (Charcot's joints) develop. Sudden and severe pains (lightning pains) may occur in the limbs or abdomen. Tendon reflexes are lost and bladder control disturbed. The patient may become deaf and blind.

Treatment

Treatment with procain penicillin 600 000 units daily for 10 to 21 days halts both meningovascular syphilis and general paralysis of the insane, and may produce a complete cure, but the response in tabes dorsalis is poor. The start of this therapy may provoke a sudden deterioration in the patient's condition (Herxheimer reaction), especially if syphilitic aortitis is present. To avoid this, prednisone 10 mg three times a day is given for 3 days prior to the penicillin. In recent years, patients with syphilis have been detected and treated, and cases of neurosyphilis are consequently rare. However, neurosyphilis presents in so many forms that a routine screening test for syphilis (Wassermann reaction) is performed on all patients undergoing neurological investigation.

In patients with neurosyphilis, a characteristic sign is the Argyll Robertson pupil, which is small, irregular in outline, does not react to light, but constricts on looking at a near object, i.e. reacts to accommodation.

Related nursing skills

The nursing care depends on the clinical picture, and the care appropriate for paraplegia, dementia or fits is described elsewhere. In the tabetic patient, special care of the feet and Charcot's joints is important because of the impaired pain sensation, and walking exercises from the physiotherapist may be helpful.

There is a long delay between the primary syphilitic infection, which may be asymptomatic, and the development of evidence of neurosyphilis, and few patients understand the connection between them. Considerable tact and sympathy are required by nursing and medical staff because of the stigma attached to sexually transmitted diseases.

PERIPHERAL NEURITIS

Many conditions, some of which are infectious, disturb the function of the peripheral nerves, and the process may be acute or chronic depending on the cause.

Acute peripheral neuritis

The commonest cause of acute peripheral neuritis is the Guillain–Barré syndrome, also called acute infective polyneuritis (inflammation of many nerves). This condition is probably not a true infection of the nerves, but an allergic response to a viral infection during the previous 1 to 3 weeks, usually an upper respiratory tract illness with sore throat and malaise.

Clinical features

Pain in the back or limbs is followed in 24 to 48 hours by pins and needles starting in the toes and then the fingers (glove and stocking syndrome) and ascending up the limbs on to the trunk during the next few days. All forms of sensation are impaired and may be lost. Flaccid weakness occurs in the muscles of the extremities and spreads proximally. The trunk, especially the respiratory muscles, and occasionally the facial and ocular muscles may be involved. The tendon reflexes are abolished. Bowel and bladder function may be disturbed. Motor and sensory deficits usually occur together, but sometimes one system is much more affected than the other.

Examination of the cerebrospinal fluid reveals a high protein level and normal cell count. Electromyogram studies demonstrate slowing of the motor conduction velocities and reduction of the sensory action potential.

The severity and course of the illness are variable, but in a typical case the neurological deficit increases during the first 1 to 2 weeks, then remains stationary for 2 to 3 weeks, before recovering gradually in 1 or 2 months.

Treatment

In the majority of patients, recovery is complete so the aims of treatment are the maintenance of life, e.g. assisted respiration and nasogastric feeding, and the avoidance of complications which will mar the quality of recovery, e.g. pressure sores and contractures of joints.

Steroid therapy, prednisolone (Prednesol) 30–60 mg/day, is sometimes given.

Related nursing skills. The Guillain–Barré syndrome, severe myasthenia gravis, acute quadriplegia due to a traumatic lesion of the spinal cord, and anterior poliomyelitis all cause paralysis of the limbs and trunk without alteration of consciousness. This is very frightening for the patient, and the nurse must remember to explain every procedure and to reassure him frequently.

Respiratory care. The nurse must watch for signs of respiratory distress; these include shallow breathing, the voice becoming weaker, restlessness, confusion and an increase in pulse and blood pressure due to carbon dioxide retention. This deterioration can be confirmed by measuring the tidal volume (volume of one breath) and the minute volume (amount breathed in 1 minute as measured by a spirometer). These will be shown to be decreased over a period of time. Another quick way of measuring any deterioration is to note how many words the patient can say in one breath. Over a timed period, the patient will be able to say fewer words with each breath.

In the event of respiratory failure, the patient will require artificial ventilation. This is ideally provided within an intensive care or high dependency unit where there is a 1 : 1 nurse–patient ratio. The patient will require intubation with a cuffed endotracheal tube initially; however, if ventilatory support is required on a long-term basis, then tracheostomy is performed.

A patient on a ventilator requires the following nursing care.

Two-hourly positional changes
Frequent vital signs and neurological observations
Frequent checks to ascertain the safe working of the ventilator
Two-hourly eye and oral hygiene
Chest physiotherapy as required

Four-hourly urinary catheter care
Monitoring of i.v. fluids, including the cannula site and infusion
 rate
Light support of the head and neck
Effective communication

Measurement of the blood gases assesses the adequacy of ventilation, and an anaesthetist will usually advise on the machine's settings. As the patient improves, he will be taken off the ventilator for gradually increasing periods until he is able to breathe on his own.

A regular check of the ward's emergency equipment is imperative. Fittings on the endotracheal tube, tracheostomy tube and Ambu bag should be standardised and all staff should be competent in ventilating the patient by hand should a power failure occur.

Positioning the patient. The paralysed limbs must be carefully placed and adequately supported. In the supine and prone positions, the legs must be kept from rolling outwards, and at all times the feet should be maintained at right-angles to the shins, the arms flexed at the elbows, and the wrists tilted slightly backwards. These postures are usually retained by pillows and sand bags, but occasionally splints are used and then the extra pressure points must be treated regularly in the routine care of the skin.

At least one bed cradle will be needed to keep the weight of the bedclothes (apart from a light flannelette blanket for warmth) off the paralysed limbs. Exercises during the acute phase of poliomyelitis and acute infective polyneuritis may increase the paralysis, but following this the joints of all weak limbs must be moved passively through the full range at least twice a day to prevent contractures. After the initial passive movements, activity against increasing resistance becomes an important part of the patient's treatment. Later, exercises in the swimming pool, where the effect of gravity is eliminated, are very helpful. The muscles may be very painful in acute polyneuritis and poliomyelitis, and regular administration of analgesia is required. Prolonged treatment may be necessary, so addictive drugs are not used.

Feeding. If the bulbar muscles are paralysed, feeding through a nasogastric tube will be necessary. There are many proprietary brands of tube feed available, and a suitable one can be chosen in consultation with the dietician. If the patient can swallow, the food should contain roughage to help bowel actions. A high-protein diet will help to reduce muscle breakdown and a daily fluid intake of at least 2500 ml will lessen the risk of stone formation in, and infection of, the urinary tract.

Bowel and bladder. Constipation and retention of urine commonly occur. Regular enemas may be needed and a urethral catheter is usually required when paralysis is severe.

Chronic peripheral neuritis

The only important infection in chronic peripheral neuritis is leprosy, which is common in tropical countries. Multiple peripheral nerve lesions occur, producing paralysis and deformity, e.g. dropped foot and claw hands, but equally important is the sensory loss. This is severe and allows repeated minor trauma to produce extensive tissue destruction, resulting in the characteristic loss of fingers and toes.

The other causes are non-infective and produce a neuropathy (nerve degeneration) and not a neuritis since there is no inflammation.

FURTHER READING

ALLAN, D. (1982) Nursing aspects of artificial ventilation. *Nursing Times, 78*:24, 1006.

CHUNG, H.O. (1982) Infective polyneuritis (G.B. syndrome). *Nursing Times, 78*:8, 315.

FERGUSON, C.K. & ROLL, L.J. (1981) Human rabies. *American Journal of Nursing, 81*:6, 1175.

LAMBERT, H.P. (1983) Management problems in meningitis. *British Journal of Hospital Medicine, 28*:2, 128.

LIBRACH, I. (1979) Still an ever present threat (anterior poliomyelitis). *Nursing Mirror, 149*:13, 33.

McCARTER, K.A. (1982) Plasma exchange in Guillain–Barré syndrome. *Nursing Times, 78*:8, 319.

McLENNAN, A. (1980) A patient with meningococcal meningitis. *Nursing Times, 76*:1, 29.

PRYDUN, M. (1983) Guillain–Barré syndrome — disease process. *Journal of Neurosurgical Nursing, 15*:1, 27.

SWISHER, C. & WILLIAMS, A. (1981) Herpes encephalitis — a nursing challenge. *Journal of Neurosurgical Nursing, 13*:1, 34.

WILLIAMS, H. (1982) A testing time (viral meningitis). *Nursing Mirror, 155*:5, 31.

9 Intracranial tumours

Tumours are the commonest intracranial space-occupying lesions. They may be primary, i.e. arising from structures inside the skull; secondary, i.e. metastases from tumours elsewhere in the body; or due to direct invasion, i.e. from nearby growths outside the skull. Each tumour will present with its own particular set of signs and symptoms. However, the following broad symptoms should be noted.

Raised intracranial pressure

As the lesion expands, it takes up space normally occupied by the brain, hence the term 'space-occupying lesion'. The pressure in the skull rises, there is displacement of brain tissue, and coning may result. Another contributing factor in raising intracranial pressure is the presence of oedema, which frequently occurs as the result of compression by the lesion on surrounding tissues.

Obstruction of cerebrospinal fluid flow

If the lesion obstructs the flow of CSF by compressing a narrow part of the ventricular system, e.g. the aqueduct, hydrocephalus results and intracranial pressure rises.

Focal deficit

Pressure on, or destruction of, adjacent brain cells causes progressive loss of function, e.g. hemiplegia from a lesion affecting a cerebral hemisphere.

Epilepsy

Seizures may occur as a direct result of a lesion pressing upon the brain, the type of seizure being determined by the area of brain affected. Often the part of the body affected by the seizure remains paralysed (Todd's paralysis) for several minutes or hours. A focal seizure is often the first indication that a person may have a tumour.

Hormonal disturbances

Patients with pituitary tumours may present with symptoms of the manifestations of over- or under-production of one or more of the hormones of the body, e.g. oversecretion of prolactin can be responsible for infertility.

DIAGNOSIS

Any combination of the neuroradiological procedures available may be used to diagnose and locate the site of a suspected tumour. Investigations include plain skull and chest x-rays, computerised transverse axial tomography, electroencephalography, visual field charting and examination of the fundus, angiography, isotope scan, lumbar air encephalogram and echoencephalogram. A fuller explanation of these investigations and the related nursing skills can be found in Chapter 3.

A burr-hole biopsy may be performed in order to establish the diagnosis. A small sample of cerebral tissue is obtained and examined histologically. This investigative technique may be employed to establish the grade of the tumour present and to provide a prognostic clue, to guide treatment.

CLASSIFICATION (Fig. 9.1)

Neoplasms are described as intrinsic if they are within brain tissue, and extrinsic (extra-axial) if they are adjacent to it. Most extrinsic tumours are benign, grow slowly and compress brain tissue without invading it. However, they do threaten life because they act as space-occupying lesions. The majority of intrinsic tumours are malignant. They develop more quickly, infiltrating and destroying brain tissue as they spread. A few of these intrinsic tumours grow so slowly (i.e. over 10 to 20 years) that they may be viewed as relatively benign.

Intrinsic tumours

The gliomas comprise a broad group which includes astrocytomas, oligodendrogliomas, ependymomas and medulloblastomas. Gliomas account for the largest group of primary cerebral tumours

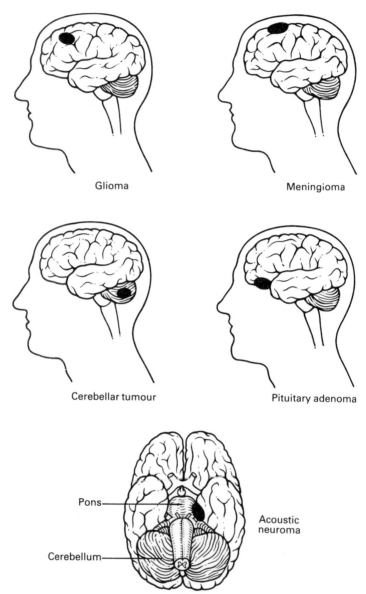

Fig. 9.1. *Classification of intracranial tumours.*

and often prove the most difficult to treat. The term glioma refers to those tumours which arise from the neuroglia, the connective tissue of the nervous system, and medulloblastomas which arise from the nerve cells. A malignancy grade from 1 (low) to 4 (high) is used to describe these tumours.

Astrocytomas

These can occur almost anywhere. Grade 1 tumours are usually found in the fronto-parietal area of the cerebral hemisphere; the more diffuse tumours of grades 3 and 4 (glioblastoma multiforme) are more difficult to localise and may be found in the white matter of the anterior part of the hemispheres. A cystic astrocytoma, which is very slow growing, can occur in the cerebellum, usually in children between the ages of 6 and 10. Oedema can occur in the adjacent white matter and this is often a factor contributing to the size of a tumour.

The presenting signs and symptoms of astrocytoma are varied and depend on the site and size of the lesion. Cerebellar tumours will present with a disturbance of the VI and VII cranial nerves, producing ataxia and inco-ordinated movements.

Treatment varies according to each case. Surgery may be attempted, although complete removal is seldom possible for fear of destroying vital structures within the brain. Radiotherapy and/or chemotherapy may be a more appropriate form of treatment. Mention should be made of the use of the steroid, dexamethasone (Decadron), which can produce a marked alleviation of symptoms. It acts by reducing the oedema surrounding the lesion and is administered as soon as the diagnosis of tumour is confirmed.

Oligodendrogliomas

These occur in the cerebral hemispheres and tend to be more gelatinous and better defined than astrocytomas. They present as slow growing tumours and in a large number of patients the first symptom is epilepsy. Total removal of the tumour may be attempted, but if not, radiation may be indicated.

Ependymomas

Ependymomas arise from the linings of the ventricles. An ependymoma is primarily a tumour of childhood and is slow growing. It is usually found attached to the floor or roof of the 4th ventricle and may infiltrate the adjacent brain. It presents with hydrocephalus, ataxia, hemiplegia, sensory loss and respiratory changes. Treatment would consist of surgical removal, if feasible, and radiation may benefit grades 3 and 4. A shunt may need to be inserted to overcome obstruction of cerebrospinal fluid flow.

Medulloblastomas

These are fast-growing tumours of childhood, arising from the nerve cells within the roof of the 4th ventricle, usually the cerebellar vermis. The peak incidence is the 6–10-year age group and these children usually complain of visual disturbances and present with hydrocephalus and ataxia. Partial resection is the treatment of choice, followed by a course of radiotherapy. Shunting may also be indicated. Chemotherapy has shown some promise, the drugs being used include vincristine (Oncovin), procarbazine (Natulan) and methotrexate (Emtexate).

Extrinsic tumours

These include the groups of tumours arising from supporting tissues, developmental tumours, pituitary tumours and metastatic tumours.

Meningiomas

Meningiomas are slow-growing, well-lobulated tumours arising from the arachnoid mater and usually within close proximity to venous sinuses. Common sites include the superior sagittal sinus, the sphenoid ridge, the posterior fossa, and the floor of the anterior fossa. Signs and symptoms depend on the site of the meningioma and indeed some grow to a huge size before producing any symptoms at all. They are more common in women than men and occur in the middle age group. Total removal is achieved in many patients and the prognosis is excellent, although recurrence can occur.

Schwannomas

Schwannoma (neuroma) is a tumour of the nerve sheath arising from the Schwann cell. Schwannomas have a predilection for sensory nerves and by far the most commonly affected is the VIIIth (acoustic) nerve located within the cerebello-pontine angle. These tumours are encapsulated and slow growing and, like meningiomas, can grow to a considerable size before detection. The patients present with a hearing loss, tinnitus and dizziness, usually having been referred to an ENT surgeon. Although, access to the tumour can be awkward, complete removal is often achieved, but unfortunately destruction of the Vth (trigeminal) and VIIth (facial) cranial nerves can occur, causing a facial palsy which looks unsightly and leaves the cornea vulnerable to damage.

Haemangioblastomas

These are developmental tumours of vascular origin which occur within the cerebellum of young adults. These cystic lesions cause dizziness and ataxia, and elevate intracranial pressure. Surgical removal is performed, although recurrence is common.

Craniopharyngiomas

Craniopharyngioma (Rathke pouch cyst) arises in relation to the pituitary stalk and usually presents with a raised intracranial pressure due to hydrocephalus, a hormonal imbalance and visual disturbances (due to compression of the optic chiasma). Complete removal is not always possible and radiation may be helpful. These are recurring tumours.

Epidermoid and dermoid cysts

These are rare and are usually of congenital origin. They are thin-walled cysts filled with keratinous debris and are amenable to complete removal.

Pituitary adenomas

These arise from the anterior lobe of the pituitary gland and are slow-growing, well-encapsulated tumours. They can be subdivided into three categories, according to cell type: chromophobe adenoma, eosinophilic adenoma and basophilic adenoma.

Chromophobe adenoma. The patient presents with hypopituitarism and may complain of amenorrhoea, irregular menses, impotence and always feeling cold. Diabetes insipidus may also be present. Eventually the growth will compress the optic chiasma, producing a bitemporal hemianopia (see Fig. 2.6).

Eosinophilic adenoma. This presents as gigantism in the pre-puberty patient and as acromegaly in the adult. The features of this syndrome are enlarged feet and hands, wide spaces appearing between the teeth, joint pain, visual loss, thickening of the soft tissues of the face, diabetes mellitus and a prominent forehead and jaw. Gradually the tumour will compress the optic chiasma to produce a bitemporal hemianopia.

The treatment for chromophobe and eosinophilic adenomas is complete or partial removal of the tumour via the intracranial or transphenoidal route, followed by radiotherapy and the appropriate drug therapy to replace those substances normally secreted by the pituitary. The prognosis for these patients is very good.

Basophilic adenoma. The patient presents with moon facies, a pendulous abdomen, abdominal stria, amenorrhoea or impotence, and muscle weakness. This particular set of symptoms constitutes Cushing's syndrome.

As this tumour is too small to remove, irradiation of the pituitary gland is the usual treatment. If the pituitary gland destroys itself by haemorrhage or necrosis, pituitary apoplexy occurs. This is an intracerebral, endocrine and visual crisis which calls for prompt diagnosis and immediate hormone therapy. If possible, surgery is performed to relieve the clot in an attempt to preserve vision.

Metastatic tumours

Although the largest group of intracranial tumours, these are not often seen in a neurosurgical unit. The most common site for the primary lesion is the bronchus, but it can spread from any part of the body. The metastases may be individual or multiple with well-demarcated edges. Treatment, which comprises surgical removal, depends entirely on each individual history, the patient's age, the site of the primary tumour and the prognostic outcome.

Other tumours are rare and produce signs and symptoms depending on their site and growth rate. Examples are chordoma, pinealoma, cholesteatoma and colloid cyst in the 3rd ventricle. Surgical treatment is employed where feasible.

RELATED NURSING SKILLS

When a patient who is suspected of having an intracranial tumour is admitted to the ward for investigation, it is very likely that he will have received some information from his doctor about his current hospital admission. The patient will be under a high degree of stress and so the nurse needs to provide realistic support and reassurance. Explanations must be given by the doctor, and reinforced by the nurse if necessary, before each investigation. The patient should be aware of the procedure involved and of any possible complications. Further information on the related nursing skills involved in investigations can be found in Chapter 3.

The general post-craniotomy patient care consists of the following.

1. The patient is collected from the operating theatre by the nurse who is going to be looking after him. She is responsible for maintaining a clear airway while transferring the patient from the theatre back to the ward or ITU. The nurse should ascertain which procedure has been performed, receive a set of written instructions for the postoperative period, and be told of any problems, e.g. the patient may be a diabetic.
2. The patient must be positioned correctly: this is usually on his side, on the opposite side from the operation to allow for observation of leakage from the wound through the head bandage, i.e. excision of a left-sided temporal tumour means that the patient is nursed left side up. Most centres advocate a 10–30° head-up tilt. The patient is left on that side for the first 4 hours, and then turned 2-hourly.
3. Oxygen is administered if ordered, and the patient's colour noted.
4. A baseline conscious level is established. Neurological observations are made and recorded on the chart. The frequency of the observations should be determined by the patient's general condition, the procedure involved, and the

patient's current conscious level. This is a decision for a senior nurse. Any downward trend in the patient's parameters must be reported immediately.

5. Intravenous cannulae and sites should be checked and the correct fluid infused. Any drains should be inspected to ensure that they are working, and ventricular drains should be placed at the correct height, as directed by the surgeon.

6. A check is made to see if there is a urinary catheter in place, and urine volumes are monitored hourly. If there is no catheter *in situ*, the nurse will need to watch for signs of urinary retention. The patient may become very restless and combative. If this happens, the patient's intracranial pressure will rise.

7. Adequate analgesia must be provided.

Particular problems which the nurse should look for in patients with tumours include the following.

Meningiomas

As this is a highly vascular tumour, close observation should be kept of drains, and a replacement blood transfusion must be carried out if required.

There may be an initial worsening of any pre-existing neurological deficits; however, this is usually transient. This is caused when normal brain tissue is contused during the removal of the tumour.

Acoustic neuroma

There may be disturbance of the adjacent cranial nerves, i.e. vagus (Xth), glossopharyngeal (IXth), facial (VIIth) and trigeminal (Vth) nerves. Dysfunction of the trigeminal nerve leaves the eye without the protective corneal reflex, and full eye care is required. Facial nerve palsies cause the same side of the face to droop and the eye cannot be closed. A temporary or permanent prophylactic tarsorrhaphy is performed and the closed eye should not be interfered with except to swab away any debris gently. The sutures are removed after 14 days. A permanent facial paralysis creates eating and drinking difficulties. Initially, a nasogastric tube should be passed in order to prevent aspiration whilst the patient is unconscious, and later to feed the patient until a proper diet is established. A soft diet is useful and the dietician should be involved in this aspect of the patient's care.

Posterior fossa tumour

Damage to the brainstem or its blood supply may lead to a transient bulbar palsy. This increases the patient's chances of aspirating should he vomit, and so a nasogastric tube should be passed, preferably before the patient leaves theatre. A 'nil-by-mouth' sign should be placed over the patient's bed for the first 24 hours, and only after the doctor has checked the patient's swallow reflex can the patient be given a small drink.

Pituitary tumours

Damage to the posterior pituitary or the hypothalamus is frequent and produces a deficiency of antidiuretic hormone (ADH). This causes the patient to pass excessive quantities of dilute urine (diabetes insipidus), the specific gravity of which is very low (1.001). If sufficient fluids are not given to the thirsty patient, he will rapidly become dehydrated. Recording fluid intake and output and the specific gravity of all specimens of urine needs to be performed. Treatment is with vasopressin, which is given by intramuscular injection in an aqueous base. The diabetes insipidus is usually transient, only lasting a few days, but sometimes it is permanent and then vasopressin may be inhaled as snuff. Disturbance of the temperature-regulating centre in the hypothalamus causes dramatic swings in temperature which must be stabilised. A steroid reduction chart may be used in the postoperative period (Table 9.1).

Transphenoidal approach. This is a new concept of microsurgery devised to gain better and safer access to the pituitary gland via an upper submucosa gum incision or, alternatively, via the transnasal route, i.e. splitting the septum to gain access to the sphenoid sinus cavity. These patients are nursed postoperatively in the upright position, and a check is kept on the nasal packs and moustache dressings for leakage or bleeding. The donor site on the thigh, from where muscle is taken to plug the hole in the anterior fossa, must also be observed.

NAME ....   WARD ....

UNIT NO. ....   DATE ....

DATE	DAY	DRUG	DOSE	ROUTE	TIME	SIGNATURE
	−1	Cortisone Acetate	100 mg	IM	6 pm	
	O_P	Cortisone Acetate	100 mg	IM	6 am	
		Hydrocortisone Succinate	100 mg	IV	Induction Anaesthesia	
		Hydrocortisone Succinate	100 mg	IV	6 Hours post op.	
	+1	Hydrocortisone Succinate 50 mg 6 hourly	50 mg	IV/IM	6 am	
					12 md	
					6 pm	
					12 mn	

	Day	Drug	Dose	Route	Times
	+2	Cortisone Acetate 25 mg 6 hourly		ORAL/IM	6 am / 12 md / 6 pm / 12 mn
	+3	Cortisone Acetate 25 mg 8 hourly	25 mg	ORAL/IM	6 am / 2 pm / 10 pm
	+4	Cortisone Acetate 25 mg 8 hourly	25 mg	ORAL/IM	6 am / 2 pm / 10 pm
	+5	Cortisone Acetate 25 mg 12 hourly	25 mg	ORAL/IM	6 am / 6 pm
	+6	Cortisone Acetate 25 mg 12 hourly	25 mg	ORAL/IM	6 am / 6 pm
		Cortisone Acetate 12.5 mg 12 hourly daily	2.5 mg	ORAL/IM	6 am / 6 pm

Table 9.1. Steroid reduction chart.

FURTHER READING

ALLAN, D. (1978) A patient with acoustic neuroma. *Nursing Times, 74*:49, 2015.
CLEVELAND, M.J. (1982) Nursing care in childhood cancer, brain tumour. *American Journal of Nursing, 82*:3, 422.
COOKSLEY, P.A. (1979) Sub-frontal meningioma. *Nursing Times, 75*:41, 1753.
FRETWELL, J.E. (1973) A child dies (glioma). *Nursing Times, 69*:27, 867.
HICKEY, J.V. (1981) *Clinical Practice of Neurological and Neurosurgical Nursing*, p. 327, Philadelphia: Lippincott.
JENNET, W.B. (1977) *An Introduction to Neurosurgery*, 3rd edn., p. 114. London: William Heinemann Medical Books.
THOMAS, D.G.T. & GRAHAM, D.I. (1980) *Brain Tumours, Scientific Basis, Clinical Investigation and Current Therapy*, p. 268, London: Butterworths.
TORTORELLI, B.A. (1981) Acoustic neuroma; an overview of the disorder and nursing care for these patients. *Journal of Neurosurgical Nursing, 13*:4, 170.
TROUT, J.K. (1977) Pituitary tumour. *Nursing Times, 73*:21, 777.
WHEELER, P. (1972) Care of the patient with a cerebellar tumour. *American Journal of Nursing, 77*:2, 263.

10   Spinal tumours

There are many types of spinal tumours (Fig. 10.1), and they include gliomas, metastatic tumours, meningiomas and neurofibromas. Classification is determined by the tumour's anatomical site and the definitions are thus extradural, i.e. occurring within the extradural space, and intradural, i.e. occurring within the dura. Intradural tumours can be intramedullary (within the spinal cord) or extramedullary (outside the cord).

The most frequently occurring tumours are extradural secondary deposits from a primary carcinoma in the prostate, breast or lung. Extramedullary tumours are often benign meningiomas or neurofibromas. In the latter instance, the patient may have generalised evidence of neurofibromatosis with neurofibromas in the skin and areas of brown pigmentation, termed café-au-lait patches: a disorder known as von Recklinghausen's disease. Neurofibromas can arise extradurally to produce a dumb-bell tumour, so-called because of its shape. Intramedullary growths are usually malignant gliomas.

SIGNS AND SYMPTOMS

Pain is generally the first symptom. It may be confined to the site of the lesion or radiate in a root distribution. Spasticity and weakness of the legs are initially unilateral and then spread to involve both sides. Disturbances of bladder function and of sensation below the level of the lesion often occur. When half the spinal cord is damaged, the patient will demonstrate a weakness on one side of the body and diminished sensation to pain and temperature on the opposite side; this is termed the Brown-Séquard picture. The speed of progression of the signs and symptoms depends on the growth rate of the tumour. Metastases may produce a mild paresis or a marked paraplegia within a few days or weeks and may need urgent neurosurgical intervention. By comparison, benign intradural tumours may take several months or years to produce symptoms.

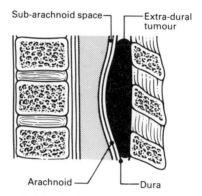

1. Extra-dural tumour

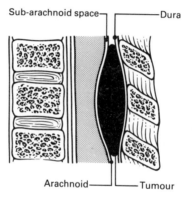

2. Intra-dural tumour   Extra-medullary

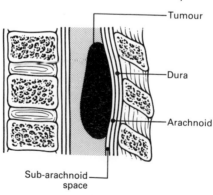

3. Intra-medullary tumour

Fig. 10.1. *Spinal tumours.*

INVESTIGATIONS

These consist of plain x-rays of the spine and chest; examination of the cerebrospinal fluid; and myelography. A spinal x-ray may demonstrate metastatic bone destruction or widening of the spinal canal by a very slow-growing tumour. A chest x-ray is required to establish the possible presence of a primary growth. During the process of performing myelography, a sample of cerebrospinal fluid is obtained for determination of protein and sugar levels, a cell count, and detection of malignant cells. A myelogram shows the outline of the tumour, unless the latter has produced a complete block in the flow of cerebrospinal fluid, in which case only its lower margin will be demonstrated. To reveal the upper border, a cisternal myelogram may be required. To guide the surgeon, the radiologist sometimes marks the skin at the upper and lower boundaries of the tumour. Myelography can occasionally exacerbate the patient's condition and ideally it should be performed only where there are neurosurgical facilities available.

TREATMENT

Extradural tumours

To prevent progression of the paraplegia and permanent loss of bladder control, an emergency decompressive laminectomy, combined with the removal of as much tumour as possible, is performed. When the wound is healed, a course of radiotherapy is usually given. If the primary tumour is hormone sensitive, the appropriate measures, i.e. a hypophysectomy for breast carcinoma and stilboestrol therapy for prostatic carcinoma, are employed. Extramedullary tumours usually allow complete removal and if the patient is still able to stand before the operation, total recovery of function often occurs.

Intramedullary tumours

These tumours defy direct surgery because it would exacerbate the remaining cord function, but temporary relief of symptoms may be produced by the careful aspiration of any cysts, and a decompressive laminectomy followed by a course of radiotherapy may improve the prognosis. Often these tumours are very slow growing, and the patient's disability increases at a corresponding rate.

Related nursing skills

Preoperative care

During the preoperative period, the patient will need to have accurate neurological observations performed. Limb movements in particular are checked and any change in the strength, movement or sensation of a limb should be reported immediately, as this may indicate a deterioration requiring urgent surgery. Vital signs, especially respirations in a patient with a suspected cervical lesion, also need to be monitored closely. The nurse should be observant for shallow breathing or any irregularity in the respiratory pattern. Frequent positional changes and inspection of pressure areas will be performed at least every two hours, along with a passive range of movement exercises. The paraparetic or paraplegic patient is provided with a bed cradle to keep weighty bedclothes clear of the lower limbs. If a cradle is not used, the bedclothes should not be tucked in. If there is a bladder dysfunction, an indwelling catheter will be inserted and should be kept scrupulously clean. Regular urinalysis and a specimen for organisms, culture and sensitivity will be obtained. An accurate fluid balance needs to be maintained. The patient may have considerable back pain and so adequate analgesia needs to be provided.

Realistic support and reassurance are necessary for both the patient and his family. The patient should be encouraged to do as much for himself as he possibly can, and the nurse should take the opportunity to teach the patient about the postoperative routine, i.e. deep breathing and coughing, how he will be turned with assistance, and that he will be provided with adequate analgesia. The patient will need to be alerted to the dangers of any sensory loss which he may have particularly in relation to pain and temperature; smoking in bed without supervision and the use of heating devices should be discouraged.

Postoperative care

In the immediate postoperative period, careful positioning of the patient is vitally important. He should be turned on to his side in the lateral position, to avoid applying pressure to the wound site, and with the body in good alignment. One soft pillow or no pillow at all may be allowed, according to the surgeon's preference and the operation site. Patients with surgery to the high cervical region are less likely to have a pillow. Accurate and frequent neurological observations are performed, with particular emphasis on limb movements, strength and sensation, and the respiratory pattern. Some deterioration in limb movement may occur due to oedema at the operation site and, usually, once this subsides, the deficit improves. Any deterioration should be noted and reported.

Positional changes and inspection of pressure areas are maintained; the patient is log rolled by several nurses (absolute minimum of three), keeping the patient's back well aligned. Analgesia may need to be given prior to turning and almost certainly routinely. Bladder function is observed, the nurse should note when the patient voids, if he has any difficulty in voiding, and the amount of urine passed. Patients with an indwelling catheter will have routine catheter care continued from the preoperative period. The nurse will encourage the patient to cough and deep breathe and to move his limbs if possible.

As soon as the patient is able, he should be restarted on his diet, eating while maintaining good alignment in the lateral position in bed. Assistance with feeding may be necessary. The patient is seen by the physiotherapist at an early stage in the postoperative period and early mobilisation is encouraged: the patient is usually got up out of bed within 24–48 hours, and gradually mobilised thereafter. The nurse should observe for any complications that may arise. These include: staining of the dressing, indicative of cerebrospinal fluid and/or blood leakage; infection; bladder disturbance, a previously continent patient may become incontinent; neurological deterioration; or respiratory irregularities.

FURTHER READING

ANON (1982) Neurofibromatosis. Clinical colour insight. *Nursing Mirror, 154*, 11.
SCHOTT, G.D. (1975) Spinal tumours—1. Classification. *Nursing Times, 71*:52, 2055.
SCHOTT, G.D. (1976) Spinal tumours—2. Symptoms and signs. *Nursing Times, 72*:1, 21.
SCHOTT, G.D. (1976) Spinal tumours—3. Investigation, treatment and prognosis. *Nursing Times, 72*:2, 57.

SWIFT-BANDIDNI, N. (1982) *Manual of Neurological Nursing*, 2nd edn., p. 125.
    Boston: Little, Brown.
TWOMEY, M.R. (1977) Neurofibromatosis. *Nursing Times, 73*:31, 1196.

11   Spinal lesions

A lesion of the vertebral column may affect the nervous structures lying within the spinal canal at that point. The spinal cord is contained by the cervical and thoracic spine, and may be compressed causing impairment of motor and sensory function below the site of the lesion. The clinical picture depends on the level of the lesion and the amount of the cord involved, and not on the causative pathology. The most important consideration is to relieve the compression which, if severe, may lead to complete and permanent loss of function.

The terminal portion of the spinal cord, the conus medullaris, lies within the spinal canal at the level of the first lumbar vertebra and is surrounded by nerve roots, the cauda equina. Lesions here produce a mixture of upper and lower motor neurone features in the legs, and because important nerves to the bladder arise in this region, disturbances of sphincter control are very common.

Below the end of the spinal cord (L1), lesions only produce lower motor neurone characteristics and sensory loss due to damage to the involved nerve roots.

Pain that results from spinal lesions may be localised to the midline of the back at that level and/or referred in the distribution of a compressed nerve root, e.g. into the arm when a cervical nerve root is involved, or into the leg if a lumbar or sacral nerve root is affected. Compression of the thoracic nerve roots may cause pain referred to the chest or the abdomen, so that the initial diagnosis may be myocardial infarction or acute appendicitis.

The lesions with which we are concerned in this chapter are intervertebral disc disease, trauma, abscess, angioma, transverse myelitis, and infarction.

INTERVERTEBRAL DISC DISEASE

The vertebral bodies are separated by discs, which act as shock absorbers. Each disc consists of a pliable, gelatinous core, the nucleus pulposus, surrounded by a tough fibrocartilaginous ring which joins the borders of the vertebrae, the annulus fibrosus (Fig.

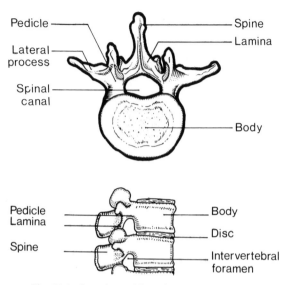

Fig. 11.1. *Superior and lateral views of vertebrae.*

11.1). If these joints are subjected to severe strain, rupture of the annulus fibrosus occurs and part of the nucleus pulposus is forced through the defect into the extradural space of the vertebral canal, to produce a prolapsed disc. The stress is often caused by incorrect lifting of heavy weights, i.e. with the legs straight and the back bent, but occasionally it results from falls or sudden straightening and twisting movements of the back. The common sites for acute prolapse are the disc between the fourth and fifth lumbar vertebrae and that between the fifth lumbar and the first sacral vertebrae. Sometimes herniation occurs in the cervical region, but rarely at thoracic level. The protrusion may be lateral, causing pressure on the nerve roots, or in the midline, compressing the spinal cord or cauda equina (Fig. 11.2).

In middle-aged and elderly people, degenerative changes occur in the annulus fibrosus, allowing the nucleus pulposus to bulge in all directions, the most significant of which is backwards into the spinal canal and the intervertebral foramina. Repeated minor injuries and, in those patients who are obese, the continual trauma of carrying excess weight, probably contribute to this weakening process. Calcification may occur in the bulges and this is called spondylosis. It is most common in the lower cervical region.

(a)

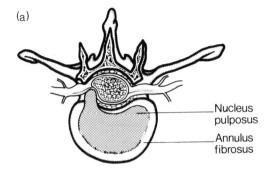

Nucleus
pulposus

Annulus
fibrosus

(b)

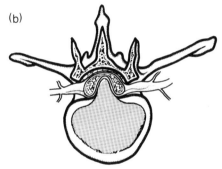

Fig. 11.2. *Intervertebral disc protrusion: (a) lateral, and (b) central.*

Acute lumbar disc prolapse

Lateral protrusion

Young people in energetic occupations are the usual candidates for a prolapsed lumbar disc. The onset of severe back pain and inability to move may be very sudden, and result from a single strenuous effort, usually lifting, or it may become apparent following a bout of excessive physical activity. After a few minutes, the patient is able to stand up, but has a marked scoliosis (twisting and flattening of the spine) due to spasm of the spinal muscles. Frequently the pain then radiates down one leg in the distribution of the compressed nerve root. This pain is termed sciatica and it may spread to the thigh and then into the outer side of the calf and the foot (L4–5 disc prolapse), or it may go down the thigh into the posterior aspect of the calf and across the sole and inner border of the foot (L5–S1 disc prolapse). There may be weakness and loss of sensation in these areas, but the patient's main concern is the pain, which is severe and increased by movement, coughing or sneezing and stretching the nerve roots as in the straight-leg raising test.

Central protrusion

The back pain caused by central disc protrusions often radiates into the perineum and both legs, warning that paralysis and sphincter disturbance (retention of urine initially, but later dribbling incontinence develops) will follow because the central nerve roots of the cauda equina are being compressed. An emergency laminectomy — removal of the posterior arch(es) of vertebra(e) — to relieve the compression and to remove the prolapsed portion of the disc is required and, if delayed, the damage may be irreversible.

Treatment

Bed rest. Most patients respond very well to strict rest and require no further treatment than a week or more lying flat on a bed. Once the pain has resolved, rest is continued for up to a further week, and then the patient is gradually mobilised. Before discharge, he is advised how to lift correctly, to lie or stand rather than sit, and to sleep on a bed which provides firm support.

If the pain does not improve, traction may be helpful because, although its effect on the disc protrusion is not known, it is a certain method of ensuring that the patient remains immobilised. Some patients may benefit from immobilisation of their back in a specially moulded plaster cast. A plaster bed is used if bed rest is to be maintained, and the ambulant patient is fitted for a plaster corset.

Approximately 95% of patients respond to the conservative methods.

Surgery. If the pain is not relieved following a trial of strict bed rest with full immobilisation, an operation is indicated. A neurological deficit (weakness or anaesthesia) prompts an early consideration of surgery. If bladder function is affected, an immediate operation is required.

Before surgery is undertaken, the patient should have a myelogram to show the exact level of the disc protrusion and to confirm that his symptoms are due to disc prolapse. Occasionally the disc is not at the level suggested by the physical signs, and sometimes a spinal tumour mimics disc disease.

Removal of a laterally prolapsed disc is achieved by a partial laminectomy performed in the prone or lateral position. The muscles on the affected side are stripped from the spinous process and the lamina is nibbled away to reach the disc (hemilaminectomy). If the disc protrusion is central, greater access to the vertebral canal is required and the whole of the lamina will be removed.

Related nursing skills

It is important that the patient rests as much as possible, and he may only be allowed out of bed to use the commode or lavatory instead of a bedpan. He will be nursed on a firm mattress with one pillow, and allowed to roll round on to his side to eat his meals. All the basic needs of the patients will need to be attended to, e.g. shaving and washing. The prescription and administration of analgesia will be required, and this will vary from simple aspirin to intramuscular pethidine, according to the patient's needs. The nurse will need to observe for complications of bed rest, and some preventive measures may be instituted, such as encouraging the patient to perform deep breathing and coughing exercises, passive/active limb physiotherapy, and the use of anti-embolism stockings. The patient may require aperients to assist with elimination. It is important that the patient keeps himself occupied with, for example, reading or watching television.

Preoperative care. The operation and postoperative care are explained to the patient by the surgeon, and the patient's consent obtained. The patient's back is shaved, if necessary, on the morning of the operation, following which he has a bath and dons a clean gown. The patient fasts for 6 hours, and an hour before surgery he is given a premedication containing a strong analgesic, e.g. pethidine 50–100 mg. Before taking the patient to the operating theatre, check that his identity bracelet is on his wrist and ask him to remove any false teeth, etc. The latter should be labelled and stored safely.

Postoperative care. It is most important to keep the spine straight and well supported at all times. The patient is nursed flat on his back for the first few hours and then turned on his side by enough nurses to ensure that the procedure is carried out smoothly. Prior to this repositioning and the subsequent 2-hourly turns, the administration of an analgesic is advisable. Small doses of pethidine or papaveretum may be given into an intravenous infusion or administered by the intramuscular route. Frequent pulse and blood pressure recordings are maintained until the patient's condition is stable. The patient's ability to move his legs and feet is checked as soon as he is awake, and then regularly each time he is turned. Any further loss of power suggests that a complication, e.g. cord compression by haematoma, may be developing and should be reported at once.

Fluid intake and output are recorded and, when the patient is drinking regularly, hourly drinks are encouraged. An intravenous infusion is rarely needed after the first 8 hours. Any difficulty in passing urine must be reported as it may indicate damage to the nerves controlling the sphincter mechanism.

When using a bedpan, the patient's body must be raised and supported evenly and this is achieved by careful positioning of pillows. It is difficult to pass urine while lying flat and the surgeon may allow a male patient to stand out of bed. The patient's back must be kept straight and if both legs are swung to the side of the bed, he can be eased into the upright position as his feet move towards the floor. The nurse must stay with the patient while he is out of bed. If a patient cannot pass urine, a urinary catheter may be temporarily required.

As the pain subsides, the analgesics can be reduced, and after 48 hours codeine phosphate is usually given to replace pethidine. Sciatic pain often resolves dramatically, but discomfort at the operation site may persist. The patient is mobilised under the supervision of the physiotherapists and with the help of the nursing staff. He is encouraged to stand and walk, but not to sit. The regime of mobilisation depends on the surgeon who is in charge of the patient. Some insist on support for the back with a corset and a very gradual increase in spinal movements, while others favour rapid mobilisation so that the patient can touch his toes before discharge. Mobility is achieved by diligent practising of the advised exercises. The patient must be taught how to bend and lift correctly to avoid further disc prolapse, and a course of rehabilitation is often beneficial. The skin sutures are removed between the seventh and tenth days after operation (tension sutures are left for 2 weeks), and the patient is usually discharged within the next week.

The best results of any form of treatment occur in those patients who are less than 40 years old and who do not return to a job involving manual work.

About 10% of patients treated surgically, and a higher proportion of those managed conservatively, suffer further back problems. Some patients suffer a second disc prolapse and if a further operation is indicated, the surgeon may fuse two vertebrae by putting a bone graft between them. The back must then be immobilised for about 6 weeks until bony fusion has occurred. Occasionally, patients complain of persistent or recurring back pain, the cause of which is not apparent, and treatment in these cases is very difficult.

Disc lesion in the cervical spine

Chronic disc degeneration and cervical spondylosis

Degenerative disease of the cervical spine is very common in the middle-aged and elderly, but only a small proportion (those in whom the vertebral canal is narrower than average) are troubled by this ageing process. Cervical spondylosis may present as brachial neuropathy, where lateral pressure on the nerve roots produces pain, sensory loss, wasting and weakness in one arm; as cervical myelopathy, where central compression of the cord leads to a spastic paraparesis; or a combination of both symptoms.

The onset of symptoms is usually slow, but may be suddenly precipitated by trauma, e.g. a fall onto the head or a whiplash injury when the head is thrown forwards and then backwards in a car accident.

Conservative treatment. Reduction of neck movements by a *collar* often relieves neck and foot pain and may reduce a spastic paraparesis. A made-to-measure firm collar of Plastizote or leather and metal is worn during the day. The head is kept in a neutral position, i.e. with the eyes looking ahead; the collar supports the chin and the occiput and rests on the sternum. A soft Sorbo rubber collar is worn at night and until the permanent collar is fashioned. The strip of rubber is cut to shape, covered with tubular bandage to enable it to be tied into position, and marked 'top' and 'outside' so that it is always worn correctly.

The collars are not discarded until several weeks after the pain has resolved, and if there is a paraparesis, it may be necessary for the patient to wear a neck support for many months to prevent progression of the disability. Analgesics and localised heat treatment may also be helpful in reducing the pain.

The compression of nerve roots in cases of acute lateral disc prolapse may be relieved by *head traction* on the cervical spine. The pain in the arm usually resolves within 1 week. The traction may be applied through a sling which supports the chin and the occiput, but this is uncomfortable and a more satisfactory system is to insert calipers through the outer table of the skull in the parietal region above the ears. The scalp is shaved in these areas and, following infiltration with local anaesthetic, the surgeon makes a small incision and drills into the skull so that the point of the calipers can be introduced. The traction weight will be 2–3 kg and the weights are hung in a series of pulleys which allow the patient to move fairly freely.

Immobilisation in a collar is maintained for several weeks after traction has been discontinued.

Traction is also employed in the treatment of patients who have sustained fracture dislocations of the cervical spine, following operations which reduce the stability of the spine and before surgical correction of spontaneous dislocation of the cervical vertebrae which, for example, may occur when rheumatoid arthritis affects the atlas and axis vertebrae. In these situations, immobilisation is important and a single pulley system is used.

Surgery. Surgical treatment is considered only in a small proportion of patients with cervical spondylosis; evidence of pressure on the spinal cord, i.e. a spastic paraparesis, may be an indication, but nerve root compression alone almost never is.

The commonest operation performed is a laminectomy opposite the most severely affected intervertebral disc, as shown by myelography. The soft prolapsed intervertebral disc material that occurs within the lumbar region of the canal is very rarely encountered, and the usual finding is a hard bony bar which cannot be removed without a high risk of damage to the cord during surgery. The laminectomy allows the cord to be displaced backwards by the bar without compression.

Some surgeons consider that it is the movement of the spine which causes the bony bar to injure the cord, and they fuse the vertebral bodies from an anterior approach. The disc space is opened and the remaining fibrocartilaginous tissue curetted out. A bone plug from the iliac crest is then placed in the disc space and into a hole in each vertebral body. The cervical spine is immobilised until fusion has occurred, i.e. about 6 weeks. This procedure is called Cloward's operation.

The patient is prepared for surgery as described for lumbar laminectomy. His head and neck are handled with great care during and after operation because of the instability of the cervical spine.

Related nursing skills. Patients undergoing head traction will require full nursing care, with all their basic needs being attended to. Additional special problems will include daily dressing of the caliper pin sites using an aseptic technique. The sites are swabbed with an antiseptic and covered with a clean dressing or small pieces of petroleum netting. When turning the patient, the weight is gently removed and one nurse is put in charge of supporting the patient's head and neck. It is important to turn in one plane, and the nurses lifting the patient's body and legs must do so in unison with the nurse who moves the head. The weight is replaced and the patient's pressure area care is performed. The traction weights must not be knocked out of line, otherwise the neck will be jarred. Sometimes mechanical turning beds or a wedge turning frame may be used if the patient is fit enough to allow this.

Postoperative care. Initially the patient is nursed flat. At one time all these patients had to wear collars postoperatively; however, this procedure appears to be less common now and many patients are only given collars if they themselves feel that they need them. The surgeon's preference will be followed in this matter. The power of movement in all limbs is checked as soon as the patient is awake, and every 2 hours when he is turned, until the signs are stable. Regular analgesics are given as described for lumbar laminectomy. An intravenous infusion is continued until the patient is drinking well. If a collar is used, it must be removed daily so that the patient's neck may be gently washed and, if necessary, shaved.

When the patient starts to sit up and to be mobilised (3 or 4 days after a cervical laminectomy and on the eleventh day following a fusion operation), he must wear a firm collar. It is not so important to keep the lumbar spine straight, but at first the patient should get out of bed by swinging his legs over the edge and rising with his back held stiffly and his neck supported by a nurse. Sufficient staff (initially nurses and physiotherapists often work together) must be present to mobilise the patient without strain to his neck; in particular, it is most important that the nurse should not pull on the patient's arms. When sitting in bed or an upright, high-backed chair, the patient's spine and arms must be well supported with pillows.

The sutures are removed 10 days after surgery. The patient usually benefits from a course of active rehabilitation with physiotherapy and occupational therapy because his preoperative state of spastic paraparesis, which is often combined with weakness and wasting in the arms, usually persists. Dramatic improvement following operations is not frequent and the main object of surgery is to prevent further deterioration.

Acute disc prolapse

Acute prolapse of a cervical intervertebral disc is rare, but can occur in young adults when lifting awkwardly with the arms stretched out in front. If the cord is compressed, the disc is removed to relieve this and a soft collar is worn for 1 month post-operation.

Disc lesion in the thoracic spine

Acute or chronic disc prolapse at the thoracic level is very rare. Both cause compression of the spinal cord, the result of which is a paraparesis with disturbance in sphincter control. If the weakness is marked, a decompressive laminectomy should be performed at the level of the lesion shown on the myelogram, but surgical treatment is hazardous because of the risk of further damaging the cord during the operation.

SPINAL INJURIES

The vertebral column and the meninges protect the spinal cord from trauma, and most spinal injuries do not result in neurological damage; but if the vertebrae are fractured and displaced, the cord may be violently compressed (contusion) or even divided. Such injuries may be caused by the spine being crushed under the wheel of a car, falling from a great height onto the feet, or by severe flexion or rotation movements (the last-mentioned usually involves the cervical region where the bones are weakest).

The injury to the spinal cord occurs at the moment of maximum displacement, following which reduction of the dislocation often takes place. A myelogram is not usually required; plain x-rays will show the fracture, although special oblique views may be necessary.

A severe spinal cord injury produces complete loss of sensory and motor function below the level of the lesion. During the period of spinal shock (up to 3 weeks after the accident), the paralysis is flaccid, but the damage to the upper motor neurones then becomes apparent and spasticity develops. There is loss of bladder function with retention of urine and, as the bladder becomes over-distended, dribbling incontinence occurs.

Treatment and related nursing skills

Much of the treatment of patients with spinal injuries is dependent upon good nursing, therefore both facets of care are combined in this section.

The damage sustained by the spinal cord at the time of injury cannot be rectified and is occasionally complicated by haemorrhage or disc prolapse, but it must never be enhanced by poor handling of the unstable spine. At the site of the accident, the patient must be lifted carefully, the back and head being adequately supported and kept in line. During transport the patient should lie on a firm surface and the same precautions for lifting must be observed when he reaches hospital.

If the injury merely involves the vertebral body, the patient is treated with bedrest until the pain resolves, but if x-rays show a fracture dislocation, this is reduced by traction to the skull (if the lesion is cervical) or to the legs (if it is at a lower level). If the spine is still unstable after reduction of the dislocation, traction is maintained until the oedema of the cord, due to the injury, has resolved and the vertebrae are then fused together.

Patients with spinal injuries require the highest standard of nursing care. They are at great risk of sustaining deformities, contractures, pressure sores and irreversible damage to the bladder because of their immobilisation, severe and widespread sensory loss, and impairment of sphincter control. If, in addition, the spine is unstable, further damage to the cord is a very real danger.

The patient should be nursed on either a conventional hospital bed with a firm mattress, a wedge turning frame (Stryker frame), or one of the mechanical turning beds, e.g. an Egerton Stoke Mandeville bed. Good skin care is vital, employing the use of pressure-relieving aids (as discussed in Chapter 17), and regular inspection of the main weight-bearing points. Two-hourly turns are diligently maintained, with sufficient nurses to perform the action smoothly. The spine must be kept straight, to encourage healing in good alignment.

Retention of urine is relieved by catheterisation, which must be performed with an aseptic technique. A major problem is infection, and one method of reducing this is to employ intermittent catheter-isations, performed initially as often as every 4 hours and then gradually reduced as the patient gains some control. In most hospitals this is not practicable, and continuous drainage is estab-lished. The urinary output, and therefore the fluid intake, must be high, 150–200 ml per hour. Any infection must be treated promptly with an appropriate antibiotic, and a sample of urine should be sent for bacteriological examination each week. Avoidance of urethral sores will be effected by strapping the catheter to the patient's abdomen in a male and to the thigh in a female.

When the spinal shock has passed and the legs become spastic, the bladder may be similarly affected, causing reduction in its capacity and automatic contraction when full. Reflex contraction can be produced by stimulating the skin of the thighs or low abdomen by pinching. The patient can learn to do this for himself and if reflex voiding has been established, catheterisation can be discontinued. A patient with a flaccid bladder can be taught to express it by applying pressure on the lower abdomen, although the additional help of a bladder-contracting drug, e.g. carbamylcholine chloride (Carbachol), may also be required. If the bladder cannot be retrained, men may find Paul's tubing, or a urinary appliance, an adequate alternative to a permanent catheter, but for women there is no satisfactory urinal and an ileal loop diversion of the ureters may be the only answer.

Passive movements

The body requires regular exercise to maintain it in good condition and if for any reason, e.g. being unconscious or partially paralysed, immobolisation occurs, the limbs must be moved by other people. The physiotherapist is responsible for supervising and treating both fixed and flaccid joints, but the nurse is only directly concerned with the latter. It is very useful to watch and help a physiotherapist as she treats a patient so that the correct method for passive limb movements may be learnt at the bedside. When regular (at least twice a day) and adequately performed, these movements will prevent deformity marring the patient's recovery of function and will minimise the extent of any residual disability.

The direct functions of passive movements are:

a. to preserve mobility of joints which (i) prevents the formation of adhesions, and (ii) avoids rigidity and fixing;

b. to prevent (i) spastic paralysed limbs from contracting and shortening, and (ii) flaccid paralysed limbs from lengthening;

c. to reduce spasticity and painful reflex spasms;

d. to maintain circulation by stimulating the muscles and hence the venous return, thereby preventing a sluggish blood flow which could cause oedema.

When performing passive movements, it is most important to treat all the joints of the immobilised limbs, not forgetting the fingers and toes. Starting at the periphery and working inwards, place one hand above the joint (to fix it) and the other hand below it (to move it). Pull the hands slightly against each other and then, unless the patient complains of pain, take the joint through its full range of movements. When in doubt about the extent of mobility, try it on yourself. Each joint should be fully extended and flexed. The fingers and toes are separated and then moved together. If a reflex spasm interrupts a passive limb movement, wait until it subsides before continuing.

Spasticity often becomes a problem and may need to be controlled by oral drugs (baclofen, diazepam or dantrolene), intrathecal injections of phenol or ice-cold saline, or operations to divide tendons (see page 220). If paralysis is confined to the lower limbs, the arms must be exercised and strengthened as much as possible so that the patient will be able to transfer himself from chair to bed, onto a lavatory seat or into a car.

Rehabilitation and long-term prognosis

Injury to the spinal cord frequently causes permanent paralysis and severe disability. The patient has to learn to come to terms with this, and a spinal injuries centre, with the skills of specially trained staff and the example of fellow patients coping with similar predicaments, provides the best environment. Assistance is provided in adapting to the outside world, gaining re-employment, coping with several problems and fitting back into society which is not geared towards disabled people. Patients will benefit from joining the Spinal Injuries Association, which provides, amongst other items, a counselling and welfare service for the patient and his family. The patient who is quadriplegic will always be totally dependent on others for his physical needs, but he must not become idle mentally. He may still be able to do some sort of work for financial reward, particularly if he had special skills or knowledge before his injury. Page-turning devices make him independent when reading, and he may learn to paint holding a brush in his mouth. The patient can also operate several machines, but he may take months or even years to become proficient in their use.

The Possum. The attachment of a possum (patient-operated selector mechanism) to an electric typewriter allows patients who are quadriplegic to communicate. Messages can be typed by sucking or blowing through a tube or by applying very slight pressure on micro switches. The machine is adjusted to the needs of each patient and, although sometimes useful in the terminal stages of multiple sclerosis, it is usually suggested for patients with cervical cord lesions or those paralysed with anterior poliomyelitis.

The paraplegic patient should always become independent even though confined to a wheelchair. He must learn how to care for his skin, bladder and bowels, and cope with daily chores about his home. The majority are able to work, although this is rarely in the same field as before the accident. When re-employment is possible, job satisfaction and financial independence must be jointly considered. Aids and modifications at home and at work, e.g. rails in the bathroom and ramps instead of steps, increase the patient's mobility and self-sufficiency, but the ability to accept help without resentment is often the hardest aspect of readjustment.

SPINAL ABSCESSES

Spinal abscesses behave like spinal tumours and may be acute or chronic. The former are often staphylococcal, with or without osteomyelitis of a vertebra and an identifiable focus of infection elsewhere in the body. The latter is usually tuberculous and causes destruction of neighbouring vertebrae and deformity of the spine. Both produce pyrexia and general malaise, in addition to the evidence of spinal cord compression.

An acute abscess demands an urgent decompressive laminectomy and drainage followed by antibiotic therapy — usually given parenterally, but occasionally in the abscess cavity — using flucloxacillin (Floxapen) 1–2 g 6-hourly for staphylococcal infection. Tuberculous abscesses may be treated in a similar manner, but good results are also obtained by conservative methods, i.e. bedrest in a plaster cast and antituberculous chemotherapy.

SPINAL ANGIOMAS

Arteriovenous malformations usually lie on the dorsal surface of the spinal cord. They may rupture causing subarachnoid haemorrhage with or without bleeding into the substance of the spinal cord. This results in sudden onset of severe back pain (like being stabbed), followed by weakness and sensory loss in the legs. Lumbar puncture reveals blood in the cerebrospinal fluid, and a myelogram shows distended tortuous blood vessels which appear like a bunch of grapes on the cord. If the spinal cord has not been destroyed by the first haemorrhage, it may be feasible to excise the angioma or to clip its feeding vessels in order to prevent further bleeding. Angiograms to demonstrate the angioma may be performed.

TRANSVERSE MYELITIS

A paraplegia or partial cord lesion may develop rapidly in some virus infections (in particular herpes zoster) and in multiple sclerosis, so that the clinical picture may resemble that due to a tumour or an abscess. If there are no definite diagnostic features, such as retrobulbar neuritis to indicate multiple sclerosis, a myelogram is performed to exclude spinal cord compression.

INFARCTION OF THE SPINAL CORD

Thrombosis of an arterial spinal artery causes infarction of the cord, especially involving the pyramidal tracts. There is an acute onset of paraplegia with a variable amount of sensory loss. This condition tends to occur in older people with other evidence of arterial disease and the only treatment is nursing care.

FURTHER READING

ANON (1982) Prolapsed intravertebral disc. Clinical colour insight. *Nursing Mirror, 154*, 21.

FALLON, B. (1975) *So You're Paralysed*. London: Spinal Injuries Association.

GOODING, E.L.G. (1982) There's many a slip (cervical spine fracture). *Nursing Times, 78*:12, 499.

HARDY, A.G. & ELSON, R. (1977) *Practical Management of Spinal Injuries — a Manual for Nurses*. Edinburgh: Churchill Livingstone.

ROGERS, E.C. (1979) Paralysed patients and their nursing care. *Nursing (UK)*, 1st series, *5*, 207.

ROGERS, M.A. (1978) *Paraplegia: A Handbook of Practical Care and Advice*. London: Faber and Faber.

ROGERS, M.A. (1979) Paralysis: how it affects movement and daily life. *Nursing (UK)*, 1st series, *5*, 203.

SPINAL INJURIES ASSOCIATION (1980) *People with Spinal Injuries, Treatment and Cure*. London: Spinal Injuries Association.

USEFUL ADDRESS

Spinal Injuries Association
5 Crowndale Road
London NW1

12 Craniotomy: preoperative and postoperative care

Craniotomy is the operation of opening the skull to gain access to the intracranial structures. There are two basic approaches: above the tentorium into the supratentorial compartment, or below it into the infratentorial (posterior fossa) compartment. Craniotomy involves turning back a bone flap, and in a craniectomy the pieces of bone are 'nibbled away'. Traditionally a wide exposure was needed to excise a tumour or to clip an aneurysm, but since the advent of the operating microscope, the bone flap and excision are reduced. For minor procedures, such as a biopsy or ventricular catheterisation, a burr hole is made, using a burr and perforator or a power drill.

PREOPERATIVE CARE

The facilities needed for the specialised investigations are often only available in neurological and neurosurgical units. This diagnostic period allows the patient to settle into the ward and adjust himself to his forthcoming operation. The surgeon discusses the procedure with the patient and his nearest relative and obtains consent. The nurse should be aware of what the surgeon has told the patient. For any intracranial operation, the patient, who may be confused, demented, drowsy or otherwise impaired, should not be solely responsible for the decision to undergo surgery.

Most fully orientated patients, like their relatives, are anxious about the outcome of the operation, and a reassuring and sympathetic approach by the nurse will help to create a more confident attitude. Sometimes the distance between the patient's home and the neurosurgical unit precludes regular visits from his family. In these circumstances, relaxation of the visiting hours may help, and occasionally financial aid for travelling may be given.

The patient's suitability for major surgery should be assessed in order that any potential risks can be established. The preoperative assessment should include: a thorough physical examination, a full blood count, determination of blood type and cross-matching, an electrocardiogram, and a chest x-ray to exclude a primary lesion or for those patients with a history of respiratory problems. The patient will be seen by the anaesthetist who will, where appropriate, prescribe a premedication and a mild hypnotic to help an anxious patient sleep the night before the operation. The patient will be visited by the physiotherapist, who will instruct him in breathing and leg exercises to be performed in the postoperative period. These instructions should be reinforced by the nurse. The nurse should allow the patient to verbalise any fears he may have about his forthcoming operation, and she can help to allay these fears by explaining the immediate pre- and postoperative care and ensure his co-operation in the frequent neurological assessments. Where applicable, a visit from the intensive care or high dependency area nurse might be indicated.

The nurse or doctor should tell the relatives the probable length of the operation ($3\frac{1}{2}$ to 6 hours for a craniotomy), and when to contact the hospital for information. The next-of-kin's telephone number or address must be checked and recorded clearly in the nursing notes in order that he or she can be reached in the event of an emergency. Before the relatives visit the patient (usually discouraged on the day of surgery), they must be warned about his postoperative appearance.

The hair is cropped closely to the scalp by electrical clippers and then a razor (safety or cut-throat) is used to obtain a smooth hair-free surface. Care must be taken to avoid cutting the scalp as the nicks may harbour infection. It is for this reason that the shave is carried out just before the operation. The wet shave method minimises skin trauma and any communal equipment should be sterilised before being used for another patient. On completion, the head is covered with a tubular gauze cap. The head shave is best performed following the induction of anaesthesia, as many patients would find the procedure upsetting. Female patients, in particular, will be pleased to learn that a suitable wig will be provided at a later date.

The patient is fasted for 6 hours, bathed, and dressed in an operating gown. If he is on regular medication, e.g. anticonvulsants or steroids, check with the doctor whether the doses are to be altered to cover the operating period. A sedative premedication is avoided because of the possible depression of the respiratory rate. The patient's bed should not be screened completely after the premedication has been given so that he can be observed frequently. The nurse should record a full set of observations which will then be used as a basis for the evaluation of the patient's condition following surgery. Before leaving the ward, the patient's name bracelet must be checked and his false teeth removed and stored in a clearly marked carton. A nurse whom the patient knows should accompany him to the theatre and, if possible, remain with him until he is anaesthetised.

PREPARATION OF THE RECOVERY AREA

A suitable recovery area should be prepared for the patient, preferably within an intensive care unit or high dependency area adjacent to the operating theatre. If this is not available, the most suitable area in the ward is used. Adequate space, good lighting and equipment in working order are essential.

The bed should have a firm base to provide good support, a detachable head-end to facilitate dressings and, in case of restlessness, it is advisable to have cot sides attached. A vomit bowl, thermometer, torch with a bright light, a sphygmomanometer and a stethoscope should be adjacent to the bed. The patient's charts, including those for recording neurological observations, vital signs and fluid balance, should also be placed on a nearby work surface. Suction and oxygen, both ready for immediate use, must be situated at the head of the bed. Additional items which may be needed include: a ventilator, an intracranial pressure monitoring recorder, ECG and apnoea monitoring, external ventricular drainage bottle holder and an electric heating blanket. Equipment for the maintenance and restoration of an airway and emergency drugs must be easily accessible.

CARE DURING THE OPERATION

The brain does not have sensory nerves which feel pain, and some neurosurgical procedures can therefore be performed using local anaesthesia to desensitise the skin and periosteum, e.g. burr holes and some stereotaxy procedures. Neuroleptic analgesia is also used with sedation and analgesia, rendering the patient co-operative and pain free. Craniotomies are carried out under general anaesthesia.

Improvements in anaesthetic technique have allowed neuro-surgeons to operate with greater safety. The anaesthetist can use controlled hyperventilation as a technique to reduce the carbon dioxide concentration in the blood. This causes the cerebral blood vessels to constrict and the intracranial pressure to fall. Controlled hypotension can be used when clipping intracranial aneurysms. Modern anaesthetic techniques have reduced the need for hypo-thermia as a means of maintaining oxygen supply to the brain cells during intracranial vascular surgery. This method can still be of value in selected cases.

Surgical technique

The positioning of the patient depends on the site of the craniotomy and the preference of the surgeon. For a supratentorial operation the patient may be supine with his head turned laterally, or he may be lying on his side. The prone position with the head flexed may be adopted for a posterior fossa approach, or the patient is sat up in a pneumatic suit. This suit is worn to prevent severe hypotension and to stop air embolism. (In this posture veins are at a negative pressure and, if opened, will suck in air.)

The comfort of the patient is important during the intra-operative period. He should be positioned carefully to prevent pressure sores and limb and nerve damage. Diathermy is almost always used in neurosurgical procedures, and nurses should be particularly careful when applying the diathermy plate to ensure the safety of the patient and prevent diathermy burns.

The scalp is infiltrated with local anaesthetic, which, if preferred, may contain adrenaline to reduce galeal bleeding, and a flap is cut, often above the hairline for cosmetic reasons. Its shape ensures an adequate blood supply, e.g. convex above the ear so that the temporal arteries are not divided. A series of burr holes is then drilled in the skull using a burr and perforator or a cranial power drill and craniotome, and the bone between them cut with a flexible saw so that a bone flap still attached to the muscles can be turned back (Fig. 12.1). In posterior fossa surgery, the bone is usually nibbled away round a single drill hole. It is not necessary to put back a bone flap because the thick muscles in this area provide a protec-tive layer.

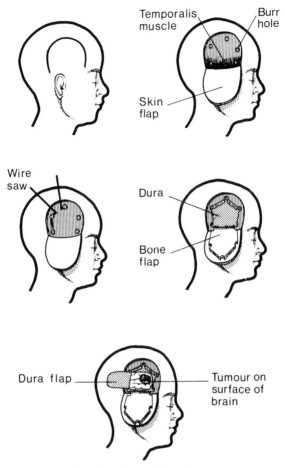

Fig. 12.1. *Stages of craniotomy.*

POSTOPERATIVE CARE

The initial 24 hours

The patient is moved from the operating table to his bed. Before the nurse accepts responsibility for the patient she should check:

a. that he is breathing properly;
b. that he is in the correct position;

  c. that the intravenous infusion and any drains are functioning (vacuum drains are usually clamped during transfer);
  d. what operation was performed and what was found;
  e. that a set of written instructions from the anaesthetist regarding postoperative care is issued.

The patient, who is usually conscious, should be told that the operation is over and that he is being moved from the operating theatre suite.

A set of baseline neurological observations should be obtained, preferably by the nurse who is going to be looking after the patient as this will allow her to appreciate quickly any slight changes in his condition. Observations are performed every 15 minutes initially and their frequency decreased as the patient improves. This diligence in frequent and detailed observation is important in the prompt detection in deterioration, such as may be caused by haemorrhage at the operation site. Delay in evacuating the recollected haematoma can lead to permanent neurological deficit or death. The nurse should check the postoperative instructions to ascertain that they have all been attended to.

Following supratentorial craniotomy, the patient may be nursed at a 30° head-up tilt in order to decrease the venous return to the head and so reduce any cerebral oedema. He is positioned on the opposite side from the operation site for the first 4 hours, to allow good observation of the head bandage on the side of the wound. Following this the patient is turned 2-hourly and pressure area care, eye care and oral hygiene are attended to. The patient can have a bed bath 6 to 8 hours postoperatively if he feels up to it. A careful check is kept on the patient's fluid balance, with i.v. fluids and urinary output being monitored and charted. The contents of any drains should be measured and noted.

After posterior fossa surgery, the patient will be nursed in a sitting up position supported by an armchair pillow arrangement, or in a lateral position with the head lying on two pillows. The most important consideration is that no pressure is applied on the wound. The medulla and nerves to the pharynx are often damaged in posterior fossa operations and dysphagia (usually temporary) results. Oral fluids are therefore routinely withheld until the day after surgery, when the doctor elicits a gag reflex. A positive reaction allows fluids to be recommenced cautiously. If oedema occurs in the confined space of the posterior fossa, both cardiac and respiratory function will be affected. Many patients will have an external ventricular catheter *in situ* to act as a safety valve, and the collecting bottle should be positioned according to the surgeon's wishes.

Restlessness is most commonly due to headache, which may be treated with codeine phosphate, or to distension of the bladder, which may require catheterisation. However, if the condition persists, rising intracranial pressure must be suspected and the doctor informed.

The physiotherapist treats the patient with breathing exercises and passive limb movements shortly after his return from the operating theatre.

Drug therapy

Analgesics

The brain does not perceive pain, and the scalp heals quickly, so that any wound discomfort is of short duration. However, some blood commonly leaks into the subarachnoid space, giving rise to a headache. The use of strong analgesics, e.g. pethidine and morphine, is avoided because they depress respiration and conscious levels. Instead codeine phosphate 30–60 mg may be given orally or intramuscularly with good effect, and often mild analgesics, e.g. paracetamol, are sufficient to relieve the headache.

Drugs to reduce cerebral oedema

Corticosteroid drugs are sometimes given to reduce the cerebral oedema which commonly follows extensive intracranial surgery. Dexamethasone (Decadron) is the usual choice, because it is the most potent. An initial dose of 4 mg four times daily is tailed off gradually so that it is discontinued after about 4 weeks. For safety, some centres use a steroid-reducing chart (see Table 9.1). Sudden discontinuation of the drug must be avoided as this would lead to acute adrenocortical insufficiency. Like all steroids, dexamethasone has side-effects, and the nurse must watch for these, e.g. salt and water retention producing peripheral oedema, hypertension, and hypokalaemia (low blood potassium) causing generalised weakness. Serum electrolytes are measured regularly and, where necessary, potassium supplements given. Diabetes mellitus may be induced and the urine should be tested for glucose each day.

Osmotic diuretics

If an acute rise in intracranial pressure occurs during the postoperative period, mannitol or frusemide (Lasix) may be given intravenously (see Chapter 4).

Anticonvulsants

Anticonvulsants are given to those patients who are thought to be liable to develop seizures following intracranial surgery. The risk factors which can increase the chances of this happening include: preoperative seizures, supratentorial craniotomy and a seizure developing in the immediate postoperative period. The drug of choice is phenytoin (Epanutin) 100 mg three times daily, either orally or i.v. If no seizures occur within the first year after surgery, the drugs can be slowly withdrawn.

Antibiotics

Antibiotic therapy is not given routinely after short operations, but the risk of infection is increased if surgery lasts longer than 4 hours or involves opening a frontal or paranasal sinus, or if the wound has to be re-explored, e.g. for haemorrhage.

Other drugs

Other drugs which may be used include antipyretics, anti-emetics and hormone replacement therapy.

Fluid balance

Blood loss during the operation is replaced by transfusion in the operating theatre. An i.v. infusion is given for the first 24–48 hours (500 ml every 6 hours). The prescription of i.v. fluids will be determined by the patient's serum electrolytes. This method of giving fluids ensures an adequate intake and is a convenient route for the emergency administration of drugs. Following a supratentorial craniotomy, most patients are able to drink on the second or third day and there should be an intake of at least 2000 ml in 24 hours. To avoid confusion, each drink should be recorded as the patient takes it. The nurse must encourage, and if necessary assist, the patient to take a drink every hour during the daytime.

The drowsy patient is at particular risk of dehydration and inadequate food intake. When a patient has a facial weakness, food and fluids should be placed in the normal side of the mouth. Mouth care is very important in both cases because retention of food leads to parotitis. The doctor is informed if, despite help, the patient does not take adequate fluids or food, and feeding via a nasogastric tube may be instituted until his condition improves. This method is often necessary for several days following posterior fossa surgery because swallowing is impaired.

Urine output is also measured carefully and recorded. This is especially important following the administration of mannitol, when large volumes may be passed causing the patient to become severely dehydrated. After operations in the region of the pituitary gland, diabetes insipidus may develop, requiring fluid replacement and treatment with pitressin. If vomiting occurs, the volume is recorded. When this is profuse the doctor must be informed, as it often indicates rising intracranial pressure.

If the patient has a head drain the amount in the collecting bottle is recorded at regular intervals, usually once per shift (8-hourly) and on its removal.

SUBSEQUENT POSTOPERATIVE RECOVERY

As the patient improves, the frequency of neurological observations can be gradually reduced. The nurse must, however, bear in mind that in a small percentage of patients postoperative complications can set in after this intensive observation period is over. If there is any deterioration, more frequent recordings are necessary.

As the patient progresses, the 2-hourly turns, pressure area care, mouth and eye toilet are reduced accordingly. Diligent eye care will always be needed if the patient has facial paralysis and loss of corneal sensation. The daily blanket bath is replaced by an ordinary bath. Skin sutures are removed 3 to 5 days after a supratentorial craniotomy and between the 7th and 10th days following a posterior fossa craniotomy.

The physiotherapist will treat the patient regularly and, when instructed by the surgeon, will mobilise him with the aid of the nursing staff — this is usually within the first week after operation. Particular attention is paid to limb weakness and, if this persists, the occupational therapist may give the patient tasks to practise, e.g. feeding, washing and dressing. Aids to help him cope with the handicap are provided as necessary.

The surgeon will discuss the patient's disability with the relatives and advise them about his prospects for recovery and return to normal activities. If the operation was for a tumour, the risk of recurrence is also mentioned.

For the patient with a slight deficit, a period at a convalescent home helps the transition from the intensive care of the neuro-surgical unit to the independence and responsibilities of life at home. If the disability is severe, the patient's stay in hospital will be long and he will need assessment and treatment in a rehabilitation unit if he is to return to productive employment.

Care of the head

The patient leaves the operating theatre with a head dressing in place. This is not discarded until the sutures are removed, but may have to be replaced if the bandaging becomes bloodstained or the surgeon wishes to inspect the wound, to exclude infection or haematoma under the scalp.

If a drain is present, it is removed on the second postoperative day. The amount of blood drained is measured and recorded on the fluid chart. When a drain has not been used, a haematoma often forms under the scalp and spreads down to the orbit causing a 'black eye'. Sometimes following a frontal craniotomy the eyelids become so oedematous that the eyes cannot be opened. Any bruising or swelling may be eased by the frequent application of ice compresses, and will disappear within a few days.

Upon discharge home from hospital, the patient should be advised about scalp care. The wearing of a wig should be introduced gradually over the first 2–3 weeks, the wig being removed when, for example, the patient is on her own. The patient should only use a very mild shampoo when washing the newly grown hair, and the use of bleaches is contraindicated. Good care of the scalp will help promote growth of a clean, healthy suture line and avoid infection.

COMPLICATIONS OF CRANIOTOMY

Raised intracranial pressure

Intracranial haemorrhage

Haemorrhage usually occurs within the first 48 hours after operation. Following supratentorial surgery, a haematoma may form in the cerebral hemisphere or in the subdural space. This acts as a rapidly growing space-occupying lesion, causing an increasing hemiplegia, a deteriorating conscious level, and changes in the pupils as coning through the tentorium occurs. In the cramped posterior fossa even a small haematoma rapidly leads to herniation of the cerebellar tonsils into the foramen magnum, compressing the respiratory centre in the medulla. Slowing of respiration may be the only change before death ensues due to respiratory arrest.

The surgeon relies on the nurse to report any changes in the patient's condition promptly, and if it appears that haemorrhage has occurred, he will re-explore the operation site as an emergency procedure.

Oedema

Cerebral oedema is indicated by the development of headache, vomiting, deterioration of conscious level and papilloedema. It may be caused by a response of the brain to retraction, anoxia during or after the operation, infection, i.e. meningitis, or reaction to radiotherapy. Treatment is by steroid and diuretic therapy, and antibiotics if there is evidence of infection.

Infection

Wound infection

Wound infection results from contamination introduced at the operation or during dressings, or it may occur when the incision ruptures and a cerebrospinal fluid leak is produced. Wet dressings suggest cerebrospinal fluid seepage and the nurse must report such a finding. When tested, the cerebrospinal fluid shows the presence of glucose. The patient is given antibiotic therapy and, if the leak persists, surgical repair may be needed.

A swab is taken of any discharge in the suture line, and the appropriate therapy given.

Meningitis

Meningitis may occur if infection enters the skull during the operation or through a cerebrospinal leak involving paranasal sinus or the craniotomy wound. It is recognised by fever, neck stiffness, photophobia, vomiting and drowsiness. Lumbar puncture confirms the diagnosis so that appropriate antibiotic therapy is prescribed.

Osteomyelitis

An infected bone flap will not become apparent until several weeks or months after surgery, and must be removed. Most surgeons prefer to use an acrylic plate when performing cranioplasty about 6 months to 1 year later.

Epilepsy

Epilepsy may follow any supratentorial operation, and anticonvulsants are given when indicated. If it is necessary to maintain long-term anticonvulsant therapy, the patient will be advised of the best way to achieve therapeutic benefit while avoiding any additional problems. The following points need to be covered.

1. The anticonvulsants must be taken on a regular basis, even though the patient may experience a prolonged seizure-free period.
2. An indication of the possible side-effects of his medication will be explained so that the patient can observe for these.
3. The patient may not engage in driving a motor vehicle or operating moving machinery, and must refrain from consuming alcohol.
4. The patient should always carry an identification card with a contact telephone number, and family and workmates should be informed what to do in the event of the patient sustaining a seizure.

Further elaboration of these points can be found in Chapter 7.

Hydrocephalus

Adhesions, scarring or bleeding can cause an obstruction within the ventricular system, resulting in hydrocephalus. The patient does not improve at the expected rate of recovery, remaining drowsy and disorientated. The diagnosis is confirmed by CT scanning followed by insertion of a shunt to drain the excess cerebrospinal fluid.

Temperature variation

Hypothermia

After a long operation the patient's temperature may be subnormal. Every 15 minutes, the patient's temperature is recorded rectally or per axilla with a low-reading thermometer.

Hyperpyrexia

Disorders of temperature regulation can occur following major intracranial operations and may be due to damage to the hypothalamus. Blood in the subarachnoid space and infection may also cause pyrexia. A rise in body temperature increases the oxygen requirements by about 20% per 1°C and a temperature above 41°C is not usually compatible with life. Prompt control of any pyrexia is therefore very important.

Heat loss is prevented by covering the patient with blankets, and in an extreme case of hypothermia an aluminium blanket may be used. It is important that the temperature rises slowly and, as it returns towards normal, that the extra coverings are gradually removed.

At 35.5°C only a cotton gown and a single thin sheet should cover the patient. If the temperature continues to rise, a fan is positioned to blow air over the patient. This increases evaporation of perspiration, which causes heat loss. If the patient is unconscious, the fan must never be directed at his eyes.

Aspirin acts on the temperature-regulating centre and can be given in the form of suppositories (1200 mg) if the temperature rises above 38.5°C. If the pyrexia still persists, tepid sponging should be performed.

Careful observation of the temperature must be continued because further rapid rises frequently occur.

Speech deficit

The patient's preoperative speech deficit (if any) and the site of the surgery will determine the extent of the dysphasia (difficulty in speaking). The dysphasia, when due to oedema, usually resolves spontaneously but if the language area of the brain is affected, speech therapy is usually indicated (depending on the diagnosis). The nurse will have to exercise her patience in dealing with the dysphasic patient, and an alternative method of communication will need to be devised. The simplest of these aids includes allowing the patient to write everything down or use a communication board.

Motor and sensory deficits

Many patients will experience motor and sensory deficits following their surgery. Any weakened or plegic limbs will need to be lightly supported. The physiotherapist should be involved in caring for these patients, providing a series of passive range of movement exercises leading to a gradual mobilisation programme. The physiotherapist may also be able to advise on any aids that might assist the patient, e.g. splints or walking accessories. For some patients, the loss of a bodily function may drastically affect their future life. They may fear a loss of employment, becoming dependent on family and friends, and a curtailment of their social life because of their disability. This can be an emotional time for the patient and he will require a lot of psychological support at this stage.

Diabetes insipidus

When the patient voids large amounts of urine (with a low specific gravity), particularly following surgery in and around the pituitary gland, then diabetes insipidus should be suspected. It is usually transient and occurs as a result of depletion of the antidiuretic hormone from the posterior lobe of the pituitary gland following surgery. If the diuresis persists without appropriate replacement fluids, the patient can become dangerously dehydrated. Accurate fluid balance is essential, with every specimen of urine being tested for specific gravity. Treatment consists of administering synthetic antidiuretic hormone, e.g. DDAVP 4 μg intramuscularly.

Loss of the swallowing reflex

Patients may experience a temporary bulbar palsy if the IXth (glossopharyngeal) and Xth (vagus) cranial nerves are disturbed during surgery or by postoperative oedema. If the patient aspirates any food or fluid into his lungs, respiratory problems such as a severe chest infection can ensue. Some centres advocate passing a nasogastric tube on all patients undergoing posterior fossa surgery, whereas others will choose which patient to pass a tube on. The tube is aspirated every 2 hours, and oral fluids are withheld for the first 24 hours when the doctor will test the reflex for normal function.

Loss of the corneal reflex

Corneal abrasions and keratitis may occur in unconscious patients and those who have impaired eye sensation, which can result from operations for removal of an acoustic neuroma. Regular eye care and the insertion of artificial eyedrops every 2 hours must be undertaken. Any sign of damage should be reported.

Periorbital oedema

Periorbital oedema frequently occurs following intracranial surgery and can be very frightening for the patient, as he may mistakenly think that he has become blind. Cold saline soaks or ice packs applied to the swollen area, and reassurance for the patient are the main nursing considerations.

Disturbance of personality

Personality changes following surgery in the frontal area can be frustrating and distressing for both the patient and his family. Supportive care is all the nurse can offer at this stage.

FURTHER READING

BOORE, J.R.P. (1978) *Prescription for Recovery*. London: Royal College of Nursing.
HAYWARD, J. (1975) *Information: A Prescription against Pain*. Series 2, No. 5. London: Royal College of Nursing.

POTTS, D.J. (1981) How can I reassure my patient if I have never been in surgery? *Journal of Neurosurgical Nursing. 13*:4, 211.

RHODES, M. & GROSSER, B. (1983) Complications of post fossa craniotomy. *Journal of Neurosurgical Nursing, 15*:1, 9.

13 Cerebral blood vessel disorders

CEREBRAL VASCULAR ACCIDENTS

Cerebral vascular accidents (strokes) are the commonest neuro-logical disorders requiring admission to hospital. Most of these patients are cared for in general medical wards, and every nurse should understand the important aspects of their treatment and rehabilitation.

The cerebral neurones require a continuous supply of oxygen and glucose and these are provided by the arterial system. A reduction in the blood supply (ischaemia) causes cessation of function in the affected neurones, and an interruption of the blood flow leads to death of the neurones, i.e. cerebral infarction. Stenosis or occlusion of the cerebral arteries may be caused by atheromatous changes in the wall of the vessels and/or a thrombus or embolus. The irregu-larity and stenosis caused by the atheroma predisposes towards thrombosis, but on rare occasions the latter occurs as a result of trauma, e.g. from a whiplash injury, or when the artery is com-pressed in the neck by malignant lymph glands.

Thrombosis is most commonly encountered in the internal caro-tid and vertebral arteries. The internal carotid artery is below the system of anastomoses at the base of the brain (the circle of Willis) and the extent of cerebral infarction caused by its occlusion depends on the efficiency of the communication between these linked arter-ies and the degree to which they are also affected by atheroma. Some patients do not develop any neurological symptoms, whereas in others complete hemiplegia may occur. Dysphagia, dysarthria, disorders of eye movements and ataxia may result from vertebral artery thrombosis if the collateral circulation of the brainstem is insufficient.

Emboli which pass into the cerebral arteries usually arise from atheromatous vessels in the neck or from a roughened area in the lining of the heart. They become lodged in the first vessel that is too narrow to let them travel further, and this often occurs at a bifurcation. Most emboli block the middle cerebral artery, and the resultant infarction of its territory causes a hemiplegia. Less commonly, an embolus enters the vertebral artery. It may stop at the bifurcation of the basilar artery, where it causes ischaemia of the brainstem and of both occipital lobes, leading to loss of consciousness and blindness respectively. A small embolus will pass into one of the posterior cerebral arteries and produce an homonymous hemianopia.

Medical care

Cerebral infarction due to thrombosis or embolism is the commonest cause of hemiplegia of sudden onset. However, some rapidly growing tumours, especially metastases, and subdural haematomas present in this way. Computerised axial tomography is now the investigation of choice in determining and locating the lesion.

The area of infarction is frequently surrounded by a zone of cerebral oedema, which acts as a space-occupying lesion. This may increase the neurological deficit and contribute to the impairment of consciousness. A course of steroids will reduce the oedema and may lead to rapid improvement.

Any other care is purely supportive, e.g. hypertension, if present, is treated with hypotensive agents.

Related nursing skills

When the cerebral infarction is very extensive or the brainstem is primarily affected, consciousness is disturbed or lost. The nursing care is that appropriate for the unconscious patient, paying particular attention to the paralysed limbs. To prevent contractures, passive range of movement exercises should be carried out at least twice daily, and to reduce calf spasticity the foot must not be supported. When a profound hemiplegia is not complicated by a disturbance of conscious level, the nurse's role is to promote enthusiastic rehabilitation. Her cheerful and positive attitude will help the patient and his family to accept his disease and to work hard to overcome or adjust to his disability. Mobility must be encouraged and the patient taught how to feed and dress himself, even though an arm and leg are paralysed. Passive exercises are still necessary and the paralysed limbs must be well supported whether the patient is in bed or sitting in an upright armchair. In the latter instance the patient tends to slip onto the floor, but this can be avoided if the chair allows for a table to be clamped to its arms, or alternatively a body harness may be used. The physiotherapist gives the patient his first walking lesson, but thereafter the nurse should encourage and assist him to walk in the ward and to the bathroom. The obese patient should have a restricted diet because excessive weight impedes recovery of mobility. As the patient's condition improves, he will benefit from occupational therapy with special emphasis on everyday tasks. If he has a visual field defect, the nurse should approach him on the side that he can see. The patient's locker and table should be placed on the side of his vision, which will be the same as that of his unaffected limbs.

There are two disabilities which delay rehabilitation of the hemiplegic patient. The more common of these is dysphasia, which occurs in lesions of the dominant hemisphere, i.e. usually those producing a right hemiplegia. This impairs the patient's ability to communicate, both in understanding what is being said to him and in expressing himself, and the resultant frustration frequently reduces a man to tears. No patient must ever be treated as an idiot or ignored because communication is difficult. The nurse must learn to recognise his attempts to convey basic needs, and daily or twice-daily lessons from the speech therapist will help the patient to regain his proficiency in speaking, reading and writing. Success depends on diligent practice, and the nurse must encourage the patient to repeat single words and phrases many times a day, praising him on his achievements and reassuring him when he is downhearted by his lack of progress.

The other disability is much less common, but may complicate lesions of the non-dominant hemisphere when the parietal lobe is involved. This is neglect of the paralysed limbs and may be so marked that the patient completely denies that his limbs are weak or that he has any impairment of function. It can be easily appreciated how hard it is to teach a patient to walk again when he repudiates that one leg is paralysed.

An important factor in the rehabilitation of stroke victims is the role played by the Chest, Heart and Stroke Association. In many areas this association provides a Volunteer Stroke Scheme which is designed to help those patients with speech difficulties. Volunteers visit the patient at home and also organise weekly Stroke Club meetings, outings and events. A welfare and counselling service is also provided.

Prognosis

The outlook for patients is variable and depends on age as well as the extent of the haemorrhage. About 25% of patients die, whereas a further 25% make a full recovery and are able to lead a normal life. Of the remaining 50% half sustain a residual deficit, but can return to work, and half are severely disabled, being bed or chairbound and requiring full nursing care.

The speed of recovery is a guide to the eventual result. If some active movement returns to a paralysed limb within the first week, then the outcome is good. Persistent high blood pressure increases the likelihood of further strokes, and is treated with hypotensive drugs.

Transient ischaemic attacks

Transient ischaemic attacks are temporary (lasting up to 24 hours) episodes of neurological dysfunction that occur in cerebral vascular disease. They may precede a completed stroke and therefore are considered as warning symptoms. The attacks are caused by emboli that travel into the carotid or vertebral arteries and give rise to identifiable symptoms. Involvement of the vertebral artery produces episodes of vertigo and ataxia, and carotid artery disease causes contralateral attacks of numbness or weakness of a hand or the side of the face, or dysphasia. The ophthalmic artery is a branch of the internal carotid artery, and ipsilateral episodes of partial or complete blindness in one eye may develop. If the retinal vessels are examined through an ophthalmoscope before sight is regained, the causative emboli may be seen.

Medical care

All patients who have had transient ischaemic attacks must be investigated with a view to treating the cause before a completed stroke ensues, and those in whom the episodes are accruing several times a day require admission to hospital. Investigations include a chest x-ray, an electrocardiogram to exclude cardiac pathology, and measurement of the serum cholesterol, ESR, full blood count and VDRL.

If the diagnosis at this stage remains as transient ischaemic attacks, then a decision has now to be made whether to treat the patient conservatively or resort to surgery. Conservative treatment consists of giving aspirin 300 mg, three times daily in order to try to prevent platelet thromboembolism. Some patients may also benefit from anticoagulant therapy.

To establish if the patient would benefit from surgery, bilateral carotid angiography is performed. Each common carotid artery is injected low in the neck, thus avoiding trauma at the bifurcation and allowing the full extent of the diseased internal carotid artery and the intracranial vessels to be demonstrated.

Carotid stenosis may be helped by performing a disobliterative endarterectomy, in which the affected segment is dissected and exposed so that the atheromatous ulcer and part of the lining can be removed. Patients who demonstrate stenosis or total occlusion of the internal carotid artery or the middle cerebral artery may benefit from an extracranial–intracranial anastomosis. This is an end-to-end or end-to-side junction anastomosis involving the superior temporal artery and the middle cerebral artery, which should restore the compromised circulation to that area of the brain.

Related nursing skills

Most of the related nursing skills involved in caring for the patient with transient ischaemic attacks are evolved around pre- and postoperative care following endarterectomy or anastomosis. Routine pre- and postoperative care as described in Chapter 12 is applicable, with the following additional points.

An accurate assessment of the patient's preoperative conscious level is important, especially for close monitoring during the immediate postoperative period. Special note is made of any existing neurological deficits and the information passed on. The patient is told that the first 24 hours postoperatively will be spent in an ITU or high dependency unit, where frequent neurological observations will be performed. The nurse should, in particular, observe for signs of completed stroke, indicative that intra-operative emboli have dislodged, and notify the doctor immediately. Routine ECG screening is performed to detect any arrhythmias, as these patients often have atheromatous coronary artery problems as well. The patient is gradually mobilised, and a return to the activities of daily living is encouraged.

If conservative measures are used, it is the nurse's task to teach the patient about medication compliance. It is important that the patient takes his aspirin regularly as prescribed, knows what the more common side-effects are, and that he reports regularly to his doctor.

CEREBRAL HAEMATOMA

Bleeding into the brain tissues may remain localised as a haematoma, or leak into the ventricles or subarachnoid space (secondary subarachnoid haemorrhage). Although occasionally produced when blood clotting is disturbed, e.g. in leukaemia and anticoagulant therapy, most cerebral haematomas are caused by hypertension and result from the rupture of a small artery, usually in the internal capsule.

The patient suddenly develops a headache (often during exertion), and gradually loses consciousness due to the space-occupying effect of the haematoma and a progressive hemiplegia that results from destruction of the fibre tracts.

Investigations

A CT scan will demonstrate the position and size of the haematoma.

Management

The majority of patients who sustain an intracerebral haematoma are over 50 years of age, and the mortality rate is very high. More than 50% of all cases die, and the proportion increases to 80% for patients over 70 years of age and for those who are unconscious when they arrive in hospital.

Survival depends on the size of the haematoma and on good nursing care. Hypotensive drugs are given to control the high blood pressure, and mannitol or steroids to reduce the cerebral oedema surrounding the haematoma.

After a period of time the patient is reassessed, and if the conscious level is improving, conservative treatment is indicated. The patient is gradually mobilised and allowed to return to the activities of daily living as he feels able. If, however, the level of consciousness is slowly deteriorating, evacuation of the haematoma may be considered, as it is acting as a space-occupying lesion. Surgical intervention cannot repair any of the damage to the brain tissue, all of which occurred at the time of the bleed, and those patients who do survive are usually left severely disabled.

SUBARACHNOID HAEMORRHAGE

A subarachnoid haemorrhage manifests itself as a result of bleeding into the cerebrospinal fluid within the subarachnoid space. There are several causes of this, the commonest being the rupture of an intracerebral blood vessel abnormality, in particular an aneurysm, and to a lesser extent an arteriovenous malformation (angioma). An aneurysm is a localised swelling arising from a weakened area in the wall of an artery (Fig. 13.1). It is often located at the bifurcation of a vessel; a berry aneurysm may develop as a bulge or a definite appendage with a neck and an almost spherical head. Other rare causes include head injury, tumour, coagulation disorders and viral encephalitis. In any one of these conditions, haemorrhage may destroy brain tissue and produce an intracerebral haematoma as well as bleeding into the subarachnoid space. No causative pathology will be found in approximately one-fifth of those patients with a positive subarachnoid haemorrhage; one possible explanation could be that microaneurysms are obliterated during rupture.

Subarachnoid haemorrhage is a disorder of the middle years of life, affecting both males and females between the ages of 25 and 50. Hypertension may also may be implicated. Angiomas tend to occur in younger subjects, between the ages of 10 and 25.

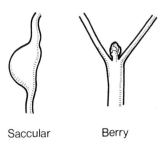

Saccular   Berry

Fig. 13.1. *Saccular and berry aneurysms.*

Most patients will experience a very severe headache, with or without vomiting, and this may be followed by loss of consciousness, although coma can precede all other features. Rupture may occur at rest or on exertion, and the sudden onset of signs and symptoms is due to blood in the subarachnoid space and the damage to nervous tissue near the aneurysm.

When examined, the patient will demonstrate neck stiffness, a positive Kernig's sign (spasm of the hamstring muscle) and photophobia. Additional signs, such as hemiplegia or a third nerve palsy, may also be present depending on the site and severity of the primary bleed. The loss of function may be temporarily increased if haemorrhage causes the nearby arteries to develop spasm and leave the tissue they supply (i.e. develop ischaemia).

Medical care on admission

All cases of suspected subarachnoid haemorrhage are admitted to hospital, and the initial treatment consists of complete rest on a firm-based bed with a single pillow for the patient to rest his head on.

Once the correct history has been elicited by interviewing the patient and/or an eye witness, and the physical signs have been recorded, a lumbar puncture is performed to confirm the presence of blood in the cerebrospinal fluid. After about 4 hours, the blood has reached the lumbar level and the withdrawn cerebrospinal fluid is uniformly bloodstained, i.e. the red cell count is the same in each of the three samples. After 3 days all the red cells have broken down to give the cerebrospinal fluid a yellow tinge (xanthachromic fluid), and this appearance will persist for 10 days.

The doctor should speak with the next-of-kin, explaining the gravity of the patient's illness, and obtain written consent for cerebral angiography and, if considered necessary, craniotomy.

A CT scan may be performed to determine the presence and site of any haematoma. Antifibrinolytic therapy may be commenced, in order to try to reduce the risk of rebleeding. It acts by inhibiting plasminogen activation and interfering with fibrinolysis. One such drug is tranexamic acid (Cyklokapron) 1 g, four times daily, orally or intravenously.

Related nursing skills

The patient is nursed on complete bed rest in a subdued, darkened atmosphere, preferably in an easily observable side room. An explanation is given to the patient of the necessity of this and of the fact that frequent neurological observations will be performed throughout the day and night. The frequency of observations will be determined by the doctor in consultation with the nurse in charge. If the patient is unconscious, the appropriate nursing care (as discussed in Chapter 6) will be given. If there is a possibility that angiography will be performed within the immediate future, food and fluids are withheld until the doctor states otherwise. An intravenous infusion may be started to maintain hydration.

The relatives are advised to restrict visiting to the immediate family so that the patient can rest. The address and telephone number of the nearest relative are recorded prominently in the patient's nursing notes so that contact may be made in the event of a sudden change in the patient's condition.

Analgesia, e.g. codeine phosphate, and an anti-emetic, e.g. prochlorperazine (Stemetil), should be prescribed and given as required.

Continuing medical management

Treatment is aimed at survival from the initial haemorrhage and the prevention of any rebleeds. The main danger to life is from a secondary haemorrhage, and the commonest time for this to occur is between the 7th and 10th days after the first. Some surgeons therefore advise investigation and operation within the first week, and some even within the first 48 hours. Others, however, feel that the morbidity and mortality of early treatment are so high that surgery should be postponed until the early dangerous period, i.e. up to about 6 weeks after the haemorrhage, has passed. It is with the delayed surgical treatment that antifibrinolytic agents have the most effective role to play.

If the patient is alert or only slightly drowsy, cerebral angiography to demonstrate the site of the aneurysm is performed within the next 48 hours. However, if he is unconscious or if there is a marked neurological deficit, this usually indicates severe spasm of the cerebral arteries, and injection of a contrast medium could exacerbate the condition and cause a cerebral infarction. Electro-encephalography may be performed to reveal the extent of the spasm, and angiography withheld until there is a considerable improvement in the level of consciousness.

Related nursing skills

Ongoing nursing care consists of keeping the patient as comfortable as possible. Bed rest is maintained, and adequate analgesia will need to be provided. A light diet, if tolerated, is offered and a daily intake of at least 2000 ml is required. Fluid balance is recorded and, because he is inactive and must not exert himself, the patient may require a bowel stimulant. Further nursing care includes regular attention to the mouth and pressure areas and a daily blanket bath.

Following angiography, a complete assessment of the arterial supply to the brain can be made. Usually an aneurysm is visible, although sometimes its exact outline is obscured. The majority of intracranial aneurysms occur on the circle of Willis (Fig. 13.2). The main sites are the anterior communicating artery, the middle cerebral artery and the posterior communicating artery. If no blood vessel abnormality is seen or it is impossible to decide which of several aneurysms have bled, conservative treatment may be employed. Previously, patients lay in bed for 6 weeks; however, they can now begin gradual mobilisation once they become asymptomatic. If the blood pressure is raised, hypotensive drugs are given.

Surgical treatment

There are two main types of operation for intracranial aneurysm.

The direct approach. A metal clip is placed across the narrow neck of the aneurysm to seal it from the artery. This method is the most effective, but it is not always feasible. If it is not possible to use a clip because the neck is too wide, the weakened wall may be wrapped with muslin or Terylene gauze.

The indirect approach. For some aneurysms, a direct approach carries such a high morbidity and mortality rate that in preference

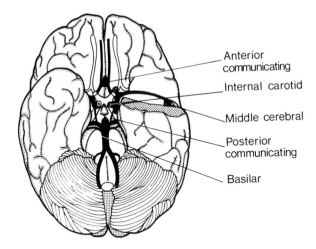

Anterior communicating

Internal carotid

Middle cerebral

Posterior communicating

Basilar

Fig. 13.2. *Common sites for aneurysms on the circle of Willis.*

an operation to reduce the blood flow and the blood pressure in the arteries from which the aneurysm arises is used. However, the surgeon also has to consider the possible adverse effects of creating such deliberate ischaemia. For example, ligation of the common carotid artery in the neck for the treatment of a posterior communicating aneurysm is only attempted if an adequate collateral circulation is demonstrated by carotid angiography with cross-compression, i.e. the dye is injected into the carotid artery on the side opposite the aneurysm, while the ipsilateral vessel is compressed. A further check is made at the operation when the surgeon applies a temporary clip to the vessels for 30 minutes and, if a hemiparesis develops during this interval, the ligature is not tied. Despite these precautions, some patients develop a hemiplegia during the first few postoperative days, and throughout this period care must be taken to prevent postural hypotension because this induces cerebral ischaemia.

Postoperatively, some centres advocate the use of an intravenous regime incorporating a blood-volume expander and an osmotic diuretic. The blood-volume expander will improve cerebral blood flow by decreasing the viscosity of the blood, and the side-effect of this therapy, circulatory overload, is compensated for by the use of a diuretic. An example of such a regime is: dextran 40 (Lomodex 40) 500 ml over 12 hours for 3 days and mannitol 20% (Osmitrol) 100–150 ml over 15–20 minutes every 6 hours. This regime will vary according to each patient and the surgeon's preference.

Careful monitoring of the patient's blood pressure and urine volume will need to be maintained.

Prognosis

One-fifth of the patients sustaining a subarachnoid haemorrhage die before they reach hospital, and an additional one-fifth succumb within the first 3 days. Subsequent haemorrhages will kill another one-fifth during the next month, and a further one-fifth over the first year. It is the last two groups which can benefit from surgery and, of those subjected to an operation, more than half will survive. If no aneurysm is demonstrated, the outlook is somewhat improved, but if surgery is contraindicated by a severe neurological deficit or multiple aneurysms, the prognosis is very poor.

Related nursing skills

The nursing care is that applicable to a craniotomy, as discussed in Chapter 12. Most patients will spend the first 24 hours in either the ITU or high dependency unit, and are mobilised 2 or 3 days post-operatively, provided there were no problems at operation and the patient himself feels well enough. There are no rigid rules and an individualised care plan for each patient will ensure a smooth and rapid recovery and discharge. Patients who have had carotid ligation performed will require to mobilise more slowly to avoid postural hypotension. The first 4–5 days are spent on bed rest, and on the 6th day the patient is given another pillow for a short while and so progresses through to approximately day 14, when the patient should be able to tolerate sitting out of bed for several hours without any ill-effects.

CEREBRAL ANGIOMAS

Angiomas or arteriovenous malformations are congenital anomalies of blood vessels that tend to increase in size. They are fed by one or more arteries and drained by several very large veins containing blood at near-arterial pressure. Ninety per cent occur in the parietal and occipital lobes, and most patients present with bleeding into the subarachnoid space. Patients tend to suffer haemorrhage at an earlier age than that at which aneurysm occurs (10 to 25 years compared with 25 to 50 years) and, because the bleeding is from the veins, the effects are not so severe. When the blood leaks into the brain substance, it separates the fibres rather than destroying them and if the haematoma, which acts as a space-occupying lesion, is removed, recovery may be good. Angiomas may also cause focal epilepsy, migraine and, if very large, dementia, and occasionally they are discovered following investigation of these features.

Diagnosis

Recurrent small subarachnoid haemorrhages or epilepsy in a patient with an angioma on the skin of the face or scalp suggest the presence of an intracranial angioma. If the angioma is large and has a rapid blood flow, the noise produced (i.e. a bruit) may be heard through a stethoscope placed on the head over the lesion. Calcification commonly occurs in the walls of the abnormal blood vessels and may be seen on plain x-ray of the skull. The presence of an angioma is confirmed by angiography, which may involve injecting both carotid and vertebral arteries if all the feeding and draining vessels are to be demonstrated. It is of value to look at, and have explained, the distinct arterial, venous and capillary phases in the completed set of x-rays.

Treatment

Surgery is used to reduce the risk of subarachnoid haemorrhage, and does not influence epilepsy, which must be treated with anticonvulsants. If the angioma is small and in a relatively silent area of the brain, so that the operation will not produce neurological deficit, it may be excised completely, but more extensive lesions are treated by ligation of the feeding arteries and draining veins. Very large arteriovenous malformations defy surgery, and treatment is conservative, consisting of bed rest until the patient is asymptomatic, and then gradual mobilisation.

FURTHER READING

ALLAN, D. (1981) Treating subarachnoid haemorrhage using carotid ligation. *Nursing Times, 77*:32, 1384.

ALLWOOD, A.C. & LUNDY, C. (1980) Cerebral artery by-pass surgery. *American Journal of Nursing, 80*:7, 1284.

BANNISTER, C.M. (1980) Keeping the lifelines open. *Nursing Mirror 151*:12, 44.

BEATTY, R. (1982) Cerebral haemorrhage — a patient's view. *Nursing Times, 78*:46, 1956.

BRANDRICK, J. (1980) A nursing care plan for convalescence following a cerebral vascular accident. *Nursing Times. 76*:29, 1253.

CALLAM, C.A. (1980) A patient after cerebral vascular accident. *Nursing Times, 76*:45, 1961.

CARROLL, S. (1979) Teamwork aids a stroke victim. *Nursing Mirror, 148*:11, 47.

COOKSLEY, P.A. (1979) A patient with mycotic cerebral aneurysm. *Nursing Times, 75*:24, 1006.

DARDIER, E. (1980) *The Early Stroke Patient.* London: Baillière Tindall.

GALBRAITH, S.L. (1979) Management of patients with subarachnoid haemorrhage. *Nursing Times, 75*:43, 1852.

HALL, J. (1981) A family concern (subarachnoid haemorrhage). *Nursing Mirror, 153*:4, 40.

HANLEY, J. (1979) Suddenly, I had a violent pain (aneurysm). *Nursing Mirror, 149*:14, 40.

JONES, S. (1982) Cerebral occlusion — a personal account. *Nursing (UK)*, 1st series, *33*, 1465.

LEWIN, D. (1976) Primary subarachnoid haemorrhage—1. The combined approach. *Nursing Mirror, 143*:3, 58.

McCORMICK, G.P. & WILLIAMS, M. (1979) Stroke: the double crisis. *American Journal of Nursing, 79*:8, 1410.

RICHARDSON, H. (1976) Primary subarachnoid haemorrhage — 3. Physiotherapy. *Nursing Mirror, 143*:5, 54.

TILTON, C.N. & MALOOF, M. (1982) Diagnosing the problems in stroke. *American Journal of Nursing, 82*:4, 596.

WALL, J. (1976) Primary subarachnoid haemorrhage—2. Nursing care. *Nursing Mirror, 143*:4, 47.

14   Myasthenia gravis

Myasthenia gravis is a disease in which there is abnormal fatiguability of muscles, i.e. during exercise; although they do not feel tired or painful, the muscles become weak. Any group or groups of muscles can be affected and their strength is recovered following a period of rest. This disorder results from a blocking of the receptor sites for acetylcholine at the muscle end-plate by antibodies produced by lymphocytes, thereby preventing the transmission of the impulse from the nerve to the muscle.

Although it can occur in either sex and at any age, myasthenia gravis is mainly seen in young women. Its course may be punctuated with remissions or it may progress steadily over a varying period of time. Two groups of muscles are most commonly affected. Firstly, the external ocular muscle, when ptosis, either unilateral or bilateral, or diploplia at the end of the day may be the only symptom for many years. However, ocular muscle fatiguability is frequently seen in generalised myasthenia and can be tested for by asking the patient to look at a hand raised in front of her. When the second group, the bulbar muscles, is affected, this produces difficulties in speaking (the voice has a nasal sound due to paralysis of the soft palate), chewing, swallowing and also breathing. Severe weakness of the facial muscles produces a snarling appearance (Fig. 14.1), and in some severe cases there is muscle fatiguability of the neck, limbs and trunk. In rapidly progressive cases, the patient dies from respiratory failure or aspiration pneumonia.

Myasthenia gravis is associated with disorders of autoimmunity, and some patients are found to have circulating antibodies. In others a disturbance of thyroid function is revealed. Hyperplasia or tumours of the thymus are almost constant features and, to avoid missing the latter, routine x-rays of the chest and anterior mediastinum are performed. Electromyogram studies may demonstrate an abnormality.

TREATMENT

Acetylcholine is broken down by the enzyme cholinesterase. Drugs

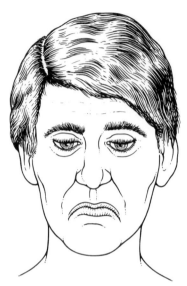

Fig. 14.1. *Typical facial expression of a patient suffering from myasthenia gravis.*

which diminish the action of cholinesterase (Table 14.1) allow the acetylcholine to work at the muscle end-plate and the fatiguability may be relieved. One of these drugs, edrophonium chloride (Tensilon), works very quickly (within 30 seconds) and is used as a diagnostic test. The usual dosage is 8 mg i.v. preceded by a test dose of 2 mg. Its effect often wears off in 3 to 5 minutes, and other drugs with a longer duration of action are used to treat myasthenia gravis. Neostigmine bromide (Prostigmine) and pyridostigmine bromide (Mestinon) are the two most commonly prescribed. Initially a small dose is given and gradually increased to the necessary level. It is advisable for the doctor and the nurse to plan a drug therapy timetable together so that meals and other events calling for increased muscular activity coincide with the maximum effect of the drug, i.e. about 30 minutes after oral administration. Many patients subsequently learn to adjust their own dosage accordingly. Side-effects of anticholinesterase drugs are caused as a result of the increase of muscular activity within the gastrointestinal tract, i.e. nausea, vomiting, abdominal cramps and/or diarrhoea. These may be reduced by giving atropine.

Injections of anticholinesterase drugs are only given under close supervision in hospital. Some patients may benefit from a course of

Table 14.1 *Drugs used in the treatment of myasthenia gravis.*

Approved name	Proprietary name	Dosage	Duration of effect	Remarks
Edrophonium chloride	Tensilon	10 mg i.v.	3–5 min	Used as a test dose
Neostigmine bromide	Prostigmine	7·5 mg t.i.d. orally increasing to a daily dose of 450 mg or 1 mg i.m. or s.c.	2–6 hours	i.m. route should be preceded by injection of 0·6 mg to lessen the side-effects
Pyridostigmine bromide	Mestinon	60 mg t.i.d. orally increasing to a daily dose of 1200 mg or 1 mg i.m. or s.c.	4–8 hours	Less likely to lead to GI upset. Longer effect makes it useful for overnight use
Ambenonium chloride	Mytelase	5 mg q.i.d. orally increasing to 100 mg daily	6–9 hours	Must not be given in combination with any other antimyasthenic drugs

t.i.d., three times a day; q.i.d., four times a day.

high-dose steroids such as prednisolone (Prednesol) 60–100 mg, although there may be some worsening of the symptoms before any improvement is seen. When the medication is given on alternate days, the severe side-effects which would normally accompany such high doses of steroids are avoided. Immunosuppressive drugs have been tried with mixed success, the most promising appears to be azathioprine (Imuran).

Plasma exchange, which involves removing the patient's plasma and replacing it with an artificial substitute, has been found to produce a marked improvement in some patients. The plasma exchange will remove antibodies and immune complexes from the blood. The treatment is performed several times over the course of 2–4 weeks, depending on the response to the therapy. Immuno-suppressive drugs are sometimes given in combination with the treatment.

Thymectomy can often lead to a dramatic improvement; however, this course of treatment can only be offered to a select group of patients. Young females, who are in the early stages of the disease and who have severe or generalised symptoms, appear to benefit most from surgery.

When the disorder has been present for more than 5 years or appears only in a very mild form, surgery is not indicated. Unfortunately the response to surgery is variable and at present there are no clear-cut preoperative conditions to indicate how a patient will respond. If a thymoma is found, the results are not as good, and radiotherapy is required.

Fifty per cent of those patients who have surgery performed will experience a marked or complete remission over a 5-year period.

If a patient has a sudden decrease in strength, she must be admitted to hospital to determine and treat the cause. There are two types of crises, the myasthenic and the cholinergic. The former is often precipitated by an infection and responds to an increase in anticholinergic drugs and treatment of the infection. A cholinergic crisis occurs through overdosage of cholinesterase inhibitors and is therefore exacerbated by further doses. Increased salivation, abdominal pains, diarrhoea and generalised muscular cramps are common features. Treatment is withdrawal of all drugs for 48–72 hours, until the Tensilon test is positive. If necessary, the different crises can be distinguished by an intravenous injection of Tensilon 10 mg, a transient improvement being seen in the myasthenic crisis and a deterioration in the cholinergic crisis.

Related nursing skills

Most myasthenics can manage their disorder at home quite adequately; however, if a deterioration or a complication occurs, then they need to be admitted to hospital.

The patient should be nursed in a quiet, relaxed atmosphere, preferably in a side room. An ongoing assessment of the patient's respiratory and general status is required, and this can be conveniently documented on one chart designed specially for this purpose (Table 14.2). It will document the severity of any symptoms and can be completed by the patient hourly. Any downward trends can easily be observed and action taken to correct these. Patients who are becoming more tired and weaker may lapse into respiratory failure; therefore intubation and artificial ventilation become necessary. These should be performed in an intensive care or high dependency unit where there is specialised equipment and staff for managing ventilated patients. It is best that intubation and ventilation are performed as elective procedures before the respira-

TIME	TABLETS	Double Vision	Drooping Eye Lids	Chewing Swallowing	Weakness of Arms	Weakness of legs	OTHER SYMPTOMS	STAFF OBSERVATIONS:- e.g. Pupil size, Counting in one breath, palpable fissure, fasciculation etc.

Name . . . .   Ward . . . .   Date. . . . .

Table 14.2 *Assessment of myasthenia gravis. This table should be completed by the patient at hourly intervals through the day.* +, *Mild symptoms.* + +, *Severe symptoms.* −, *Absence of symptoms.*

tory crisis occurs, rather than after, in a rushed emergency situation.

The department to which the patient is to be transferred should be given as much notice as possible, and also information regarding the patient's condition. An explanation is given to the patient of what is happening and why it is necessary to transfer him to another ward.

The following points should be considered when nursing ventilated patients.

Two-hourly positional changes
Light support for the patient's head and neck
Four-hourly eye and oral hygiene
Four-hourly urinary catheter care (where applicable)
Supervision of i.v. fluids including the cannula site and infusion rate
Frequent vital signs and neurological observations
Frequent checks to ascertain safe working of the ventilator
Administration of sedation as required
Neuromuscular blocking drugs such as pancuronium bromide (Pavulon) must be avoided.

As the patient's respiratory function improves, he can be weaned from the ventilator and returned to his own ward.

The patient must have suction and oxygen in good working order at his bedside and must be given encouragement and reassurance. Some patients will dwell on what has happened to them and worry that it might recur.

Medication must be given at the correct times and the opportunity should be taken to discuss the drug regime so that the patient will find it easier to manage his drugs at home. In those patients who already have a well-established drug timetable, it is necessary to maintain that schedule even though it may not fit in with the hospital medicine rounds. If more convenient, the patient can be given his medication to take as it suits him, provided that precautions are taken to prevent any other patients from taking the tablets by mistake.

Myasthenics will display some degree of bulbar weakness, which may necessitate passing a nasogastric tube and feeding the patient with a liquid diet, preferably one of the proprietary foods which are available, or the patient may manage a soft diet if taken slowly and carefully. Some means of keeping the food hot will be necessary if it takes the patient a prolonged time to eat it. The dietician should be consulted and the patient's diet discussed.

The patient's day should be planned to include regular rest periods, and he should be educated to avoid particularly stressful situations and getting involved in arguments or heated discussions.

The typical inexpressive face of the myasthenic patient may lead to the impression that he is mentally dull and stupid. This is an erroneous assumption to make, and the more isolated the patient becomes socially, the more difficult it is to treat the disorder. Ward staff can, by their example, encourage other patients to overcome their initial reticence towards the myasthenic patient. The newly diagnosed patient will have many questions to ask and the nurse should answer them as honestly as possible, referring to the doctor and other personnel where appropriate.

PATIENT TEACHING

Patient teaching is an ongoing process and starts on the first day of admission to hospital. Familiarising the patient with his drugs, the most effective times to take them, and the common side-effects, will assist in obtaining the optimum value in treatment. Patented drugs should not be taken without first consulting the doctor. An optimistic outlook should be maintained: many patients will have only very mild or infrequent symptoms for many years. Advice should be given on diet and life-style (as already outlined) and involvement in a self-help organisation such as the British Society of Myasthenics will be of benefit.

Some patients will feel more secure carrying a card detailing their illness in the event of sudden crisis. Medic-Alert jewellery is a useful alternative.

FURTHER READING

ALLAN, D. (1982) Nursing aspects of artificial ventilation. *Nursing Times, 78*:24, 1006.

ANCHIE, T. (1981) Plasmapheresis as a treatment for myasthenia gravis. *Journal of Neurosurgical Nursing, 13*:1, 23.

BARRY, L. (1982) The patient with myasthenia gravis really needs you. *Nursing (US), 12*:7, 50.

GOODGER, E. (1981) Myasthenia gravis: life-transforming treatments. *Nursing Mirror, 153*:11, 40.

HROVATH, M. (1982) Myasthenia gravis: a nursing approach. *Journal of Neuro-surgical Nursing, 14*:1, 7.
SIMPSON, J.A. (1982) Myasthenia gravis. *The Practitioner, 226*:1368, 1045.

USEFUL ADDRESS

British Association of Myasthenics
91 Cartlow Hall
Oswaldtwistle
Lancashire

15 Multiple sclerosis

Multiple sclerosis is a demyelinating disorder of the nervous system in which there is sporadic destruction of the myelin sheath, by an unknown agent (Fig. 15.1). The lesions form plaques and are disseminated in time and space throughout the central nervous system. The resultant episodes of neurological disturbances may completely resolve, but histological evidence of the demyelination always remains. The disease pattern consists of a series of exacerbations, necessitating admission to hospital for supportive treatment, followed by a remission of varying degrees. However, with each attack the neurological impairment increases, demonstrating a pattern of progressive deterioration. Each of the attacks varies in duration, intensity and frequency, and no two patients will demonstrate the same pattern.

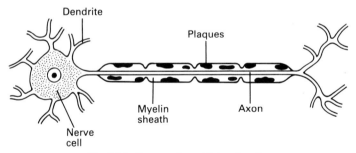

Fig. 15.1. *Neurone in multiple sclerosis.*

It is a disease commencing in early adulthood, the first attack manifesting itself between the ages of 20 and 30, and found more often in women than men. The disease is not hereditary, but the chances of a blood relative of a sufferer contracting the disease are 10 to 15 times higher than those for the general population. The disease will strike 40–50 people per 100 000 of the population of the UK, and there is a higher incidence of the disease in temperate climates than in tropical regions. Even people who move from a high-risk area to a low-risk area do not decrease their chances of contracting the disorder. The reasons for this are as yet unknown.

The cause of multiple sclerosis has not yet been established. However, extensive research has indicated that a disorder of the autoimmune system may be responsible, and those patients suffering from multiple sclerosis have an increased susceptibility to viral infections.

SIGNS AND SYMPTOMS

The clinical history will be variable, and some or all of the following features may be present.

1. Blurring of the vision, which may be associated with pain on movement of the eye. This is termed retrobulbar neuritis.
2. Diplopia (blurring of vision and diplopia can often be the first indication of multiple sclerosis).
3. Severe sensory disturbances resulting in loss of muscle control. The patient may notice that he has become increasingly clumsy.
4. Tingling, stiffness or heaviness of one or both legs, and later spasticity, may occur making walking difficult.
5. Bladder disturbances. There may be frequency or hesitancy of micturition. Some patients will present with an acute retention of urine.
6. Ataxia due to cerebellar and brainstem lesions. The gait becomes broadbased and unsteady, and when the patient attempts to use his hands, he is impeded by an uncontrollable jerkiness, i.e. intention tremor. Speech becomes slurred and irregular, with the syllables pronounced separately, e.g. hip-po-pot-am-mus. This is termed 'scanning speech' or cerebellar dysarthria. Nystagmus is a common finding, but rarely produces symptoms.
7. Fatigue, which is out of proportion to the function performed by the patient.
8. Intellectual and mood disturbances indicate involvement of the frontal lobes. Euphoria and depression are both common.
9. Impotence.

DIAGNOSIS

There is no definitive laboratory test that will immediately confirm the diagnosis of multiple sclerosis. Suspicion is raised if the patient presents with any of the above clinical features in a exacerbation/remission pattern, although this can take several years to establish. It should always be borne in mind that any of the symptoms can be caused by other disease processes, and so a differential diagnosis needs to be established, e.g. ataxia may be due to a cerebellar tumour.

Examination of the cerebrospinal fluid will determine the presence of oliglonal bands in approximately 90% of those patients with multiple sclerosis. When ocular symptoms occur, there may be delayed visual-evoked responses demonstrated as explained in Chapter 3.

MEDICAL TREATMENT

There is no specific treatment for multiple sclerosis. Many drugs have been tried, and the commonest in use today is adrenocorticotrophic hormone (ACTH). It is thought to lessen the severity of an acute attack and is only prescribed during this time. Long-term use of steroids has been shown to be ineffective. The dosage is 80 units per day intramuscularly, gradually reduced over a 4–6-week period. Side-effects may consist of hypersensitivity reactions, a retention of sodium and a depletion of potassium, and an aggravation of current infection, hypertension or diabetes. It may be necessary to administer an antacid, diuretics and/or a potassium supplement during the course of ACTH administration. Prednisolone (Prednesol) may also be used during a relapse.

Complete bed rest is provided during the early stages of the acute stage, with brief range of movement exercises being performed by the physiotherapist. It is important that the patient is not given unrealistic goals to achieve, which will place him under stress and from which he will become over-fatigued. Exercising in the gymnasium, or a cool swimming pool, will help achieve maximum mobility from both affected and unaffected limbs.

Two types of dietary therapy have become popular: the first, a gluten-free diet, came about because it was thought that the incidence of multiple sclerosis was low in those countries where people eat little or no wheat. However, this has proved to be erroneous, and there is no scientific evidence to prove that a gluten-free diet will cure or even modify multiple sclerosis. The second dietary measure involves the polyunsaturated fats in the form of lineolic acid, which is found in the myelin sheath. In patients with multiple sclerosis, low levels of polyunsaturated fats were detected in the blood cells and plasma as compared with healthy people. A modified dietary intake consisting of a daily dose of 30 ml of sunflower seed oil and a reduction in animal fats will, in theory, redress the balance. Unfortunately the diet has not been a resounding success; some patients will benefit, in the form of a milder relapse, but for many the diet makes no difference to the course of their illness.

Overweight patients will need to go on a reducing diet, and will need advice on how to adhere to an appropriate weight.

Drug therapy which may benefit the patient is supportive only. Those patients suffering from urgency of micturition may respond to the use of an anticholinergic drug such as emepronium (Cetiprin) 100–200 mg thrice daily, which will reduce bladder muscle tone and may control urinary frequency. Conversely, if there is hesitation in micturition, then a cholinergic drug such as distigmine bromide (Ubretid) 5 mg twice daily, which will contract the voluntary muscles of the bladder, can be used. Bladder infections are common, and prescription of the appropriate antibiotic will be required. A reduction in spasticity of the limbs may be achieved with the use of baclofen (Lioresal) 5 mg daily, rising to a maximum of 60 mg.

If the patient has a severe spasticity which does not respond to drugs and physiotherapy, then an intrathecal injection of phenol at the appropriate level may be considered. One of the undesirable side-effects of this procedure can be a loss of bladder control, therefore it is only performed on specially selected cases, e.g. young patients with very severe spasticity or those patients who may already have lost their bladder control.

Related nursing skills

The techniques of nursing care of the paraplegic patient become applicable in advanced cases of multiple sclerosis (see Chapter 17). In the early stages the patient will be physically independent, but mentally he may need a lot of reassurance, especially if he knows his diagnosis.

Bladder care

Bladder care is of particular importance because interference with micturition is very common. As the patient's bladder control deteriorates, incontinence with overflow, and subsequent urinary tract infections, may occur. If a male patient becomes permanently incontinent, a urinary appliance may help. A sheath is placed over the penis and the urine collected in a bag, which is usually strapped to the patient's leg. Difficulties in keeping the apparatus in position and clean enough to prevent repeated urinary infections may occur. While one appliance is in use, the other should be washed thoroughly in hot soapy water, dipped in a disinfectant, rinsed and hung up to dry. Catheterisation, which is needed in female patients with no bladder control, may also be the only answer for male sufferers; however, this final step should be avoided for as long as possible because of the risks attached to a permanent indwelling catheter.

Urinary tract infections can be kept to a minimum if a high fluid intake is maintained and recatheterisation is performed as an aseptic technique. Where the catheter enters, the urethra must be swabbed clean with sterile normal saline twice a day.

Strict cleanliness in emptying the full catheter bag is also of great importance, and it is preferable to use a new bag with attached tubing on each occasion. It is not agreed whether spigotting off a catheter helps retain some bladder control or merely encourages infection. From the patient's point of view, it is less cumbersome to have a spigotted catheter by day rather than one attached to a urine bag, as is necessary at night. If an emptying response can be established, the patient can control his micturition. The desired effect is not instantaneous, but achieved by diligent practice, and daily residual catheterisations are continued until the bladder is being emptied satisfactorily. A successful routine replaces permanent catheterisation.

Having stated the risks and necessary precautions that permanent catheterisation involves, the advantages must not be overlooked. Incontinence is socially embarrassing and very damaging to the skin. Thus the patient is usually very pleased when he is allowed to be permanently dry. A welcome reduction in the amount of laundry is another important advantage when patients are being nursed at home.

Bowel care

Each patient needs to establish his own routine, and this should be adhered to whether he is at home or in hospital. Regular aperients and a rectal stimulant (suppositories or an enema) once or twice a week will usually be effective. If this bowel evacuation rhythm is instituted in hospital, the patient may be less likely to dose himself to achieve regularity in bowel habits, which can easily become an obsession. A high fluid intake and a diet containing plenty of roughage help avoid constipation. Some patients cannot evacuate their bowels, and in such cases a manual removal of faeces by the nurse will be required. To soften the stool, an olive-oil retention enema may be given.

Care of the skin

The patient's skin becomes very vulnerable to breakdown because of the sensory loss experienced in multiple sclerosis. Prevention is very much the keyword, with the patient being turned or moved every 2 hours, or more frequently as required. It should be borne in mind that the patient who is sitting up in a chair will need to have his position changed just as frequently as he would if he were in bed. Should the patient show any signs of developing a pressure sore, then the sooner this is recognised and effectively treated, the easier it is to restore the integrity of the skin. The treatment of pressure sores is discussed in the chapter on care of the paralysed patient (Chapter 17).

Physiotherapy

The advice of the physiotherapist should be sought at an early stage in order that an effective plan of treatment can be started.

Psychological care

At some point the patient will need to be told of the diagnosis, and it is hoped that the patient and doctor can sit down together and discuss the full implications of the disorder. A keen and enthusiastic frame of mind is more conducive to the patient's rehabilitation; however, not everyone will accept the diagnosis calmly and quietly. Once the doctor has left and the patient has had time to think over what has been said, it is then he will often turn to the nurse for advice and support. He may display bewilderment, anger or frustration at his situation, and it is important that the nurse remains calm and confident and talks to the patient, answering as many of his questions as honestly as possible.

A time will come when the patient needs to come to terms with his situation, and he may display one of several attitudes.

1. Complete denial. The patient may deny that the disorder exists, despite being told of the diagnosis, and he may even display an attitude of euphoria inappropriate to the situation.
2. Regression. The patient will adopt an attitude of complete helplessness, feigning invalidity when he is quite capable of certain physical functions. This invalidity may be extended to include avoiding talking to other individuals such as nurses and fellow patients.
3. Depression and anxiety states. The patient may express feelings about loss of stature within the community and as a breadwinner. Very severe depression and anxiety states can occur as the patient ruminates about his future, based on his limited knowledge of the disease. Some patients may express suicidal thoughts, which need to be taken seriously.

PATIENT TEACHING

The patient and his closest relative will require advice and education about his disorder. Points that need to be covered include the following.

1. Advice on care of the bladder, bowels and skin. The patient's relatives will need to be taught basic nursing procedures, e.g. how to transfer the patient safely from his bed to his chair.
2. The medication regime is explained to the patient and his relatives. The various drugs being used and possible side-effects need to be outlined, as well as dosages and times of administration.
3. The patient should be encouraged to lead as full a life as possible, both at work and within the family. Those patients who go out to work should be urged to continue their occupation, and where transport becomes difficult, a hand-controlled car will be useful.

4. Patients should be made aware of the provisions of the Chronically Sick and Disabled Persons Act 1970. Its main points cover providing assistance with adaptations to the home in order to accommodate a wheelchair; provisions for toilet and bathroom aids; help with transport and holidays; provisions for access to public buildings; access to public toilets; and the issue of a badge allowing additional parking privileges. The act also states that young, chronic sick patients should be accommodated, where necessary, in a Young Chronic Sick Unit and not in a geriatric ward.

5. Financial assistance can be obtained in a variety of forms. Those patients unable to work may qualify for Invalidity Benefit, with additional supplements for dependent family members. A mobility allowance can be paid out for those patients who are sufficiently incapacitated to prevent them walking any distance. The patient and his family may be entitled to free medications, dental treatment and school meals if their income is low. An attendance allowance may be paid to the spouse of a disabled person who requires constant care and attention. Rent and rates rebates may also be refunded. The services of the medical social worker should be used to untangle the maze of benefits and allowances, as many patients are unaware of what they are entitled to claim for.

6. Sexual problems: many men will experience impotence and suffer a great deal of frustration as a result of this. Women can, in many cases, become pregnant; however, advice should be sought from their general practitioner before conception occurs. Sexual problems need to be discussed openly with the partner involved, and outside help can be sought from Sexual and Personal Relationships of the Disabled (SPOD), a voluntary organisation set up to advise on these types of problems.

The patient would find it advantageous to join the Multiple Sclerosis Society. Its network of local branches can provide support and advice on all matters related to the disorder, and also a chance to talk and meet with fellow sufferers. Crack Multiple Sclerosis is a group specifically designed for the younger sufferer.

The outlook for multiple sclerosis patients is variable: some advance to a severe degree of disability, while others may remain relatively symptom free for many years. Until a cure is found, skilled nursing will continue to form the basis of the patient's care.

FURTHER READING

CONROY, R. (1982) Multiple sclerosis: a slow decline. *Nursing Mirror 155*:11, 62.

COOKSLEY, P.A. (1979) A patient with multiple sclerosis. *Nursing Times, 75*:45, 1925.

DAVIDSON, D.L.W. & LENMAN, J.A.R. (1981) *Neurological Therapeutics*, p. 117. London: Pitman Medical.

DAVIES, N. (1980) Both sides of the sheet (multiple sclerosis). *Nursing Mirror, 150*:18, 50.

DICK, G., KELLY, R., DAVISON, A.N., BOYER, A., FEENEY, S., FINCH, K., FLYNN, M., LIMOUZE, B., NOSEWORTHY, S.J. & CONNELL, H.J. (1976) A symposium on multiple sclerosis. *Nursing Mirror, 143*:6, 45.

GOLD, P. (1981) A credit to the family (multiple sclerosis). *Nursing Mirror, 153*:22, 44.

HALL, M. (1978) Fighting an unpredictable enemy (multiple sclerosis). *Nursing Mirror, 147*:18, 27.

KINLEY, A.E., SLATER, R.J., YEARWOOD, A.C., PLANK, C., PRICE, G., CATANZARO, M., McDONNELL, M., HENTGEN, J., HOLLAND, N., LEVISON, P.W. & WEEKS, C.C. (1980) Multiple sclerosis. *American Journal of Nursing, 80*:2, 273.

MAGGS, A. (1981) Multiple sclerosis—1. *Nursing Times, 77*:10, 414.

MAGGS, A. (1981) Multiple sclerosis—2. *Nursing Times, 77*:11, 464.

MATHEWS, B. (1983) Multiple sclerosis. *The Practitioner, 227*:1377, 365.

RAWSON, M. (1980) Cause and cure unknown (multiple sclerosis). *Nursing Mirror, 150*:18, 48.

WALFORD, J. (1983) Helping patients with multiple sclerosis. *The Practitioner, 227*:1377, 484.

USEFUL ADDRESSES

Multiple Sclerosis Society
286 Munster Road
London SW6 6AP

Sexual and Personal Relationships of the Disabled
The Diorama
14 Peto Place
London NW1 4DT

Royal Association for Disability and Rehabilitation
25 Mortimer Street
London W1H 8AB

Disabled Living Foundation
346 Kensington High Street
London W1N 8NS

16   Parkinson's disease

Parkinson's disease (paralysis agitans) is due to the degeneration of the dopamine-containing neurones in the brainstem and basal ganglia, the aetiology of which, in most cases, is unknown. This process usually begins between the ages of 50 and 60 years, affects men and women equally, and is the commonest cause of progressive neurological disability in older patients. The main features are tremor, rigidity and slowness of movement. Idiopathic parkinsonism is the most common type. However, some patients who contracted encephalitis lethargica in the 1916–28 epidemic developed post-encephalitic parkinsonism as a sequel, and are now in the 65–75-year age group, and almost all are cared for in long-stay institutions. No new outbreaks of post-encephalitic parkinsonism have been noted.

Parkinsonian symptoms can be induced in patients taking large doses of phenothiazine (a major tranquilliser), and in these cases the drug is withdrawn completely or, where this is not practical, additional drugs are given to combat the extrapyramidal symptoms.

CLINICAL FEATURES

Tremor

The parkinsonian tremor is complex, rapid and most marked at rest. The pill-rolling action of the fingers and the alternating rotation of the wrists diminish or disappear on voluntary movement. The tremor is often confined to one limb or one side of the body for several months or years before becoming bilateral.

Rigidity

The tone in the limbs is increased. Passive limb movements reveal a lead-pipe (smooth) or cogwheel (jerky) rigidity. The normal smoothness of the movements is made jerky when a tremor is superimposed.

Bradykinesia

The term bradykinesia is used to describe slowness in initiating movements, and is most noticeable in the lack of gestures and facial expression. The posture achieved by a movement may be maintained for an abnormally long period, e.g. a smile may persist many seconds (Cheshire cat smile).

Postural abnormalities

The parkinsonian posture and gait are characteristic. The back and limbs are flexed and the arms are held into the chest. The patient is slow to initiate walking and stands shuffling his feet before moving with short steps. His body leans forward and his arms are held stiffly by his side. Frequently the pace of walking increases (festination) and the patient may be unable to stop until he falls or collides with an immobile object. When standing, a push may precipitate this uncontrollable trotting and the patient may move forwards (propulsion) or backwards (retropulsion).

Associated with these features, the patient notices increasing difficulty in fine movements, e.g. fastening buttons, handling a knife and fork. His writing becomes small and uneven. The actions of rising from a chair or turning over in bed prove more and more difficult. The voice is monotonous, weak and tends to peter out as the patient talks. Sentences often become an unintelligible run of words. The mask-like face suggests that the patient is stupid, but his mental state is normal, although depression may accompany the disease. Constipation and bladder disturbances are common features.

TREATMENT

It is essential to keep the patient as mobile as possible. Each day the limbs are put through their full range of use, and the combined efforts of physiotherapy, nursing and occupational therapy staff help to prevent hypostatic pneumonia, reduce disability and encourage independence.

Medical treatment is mainly by drugs that reduce tremor, rigidity and bradykinesia. The most effective drug therapy is with L-dopa, given as an oral preparation of 250 mg two or three times daily, increasing gradually to 2–3 g daily. L-Dopa is converted to dopamine, which is a neurotransmitter (chemical mediator at a synapse). The amount of dopamine is greatly reduced in the basal ganglia of patients with Parkinson's disease, and many improve quite dramatically following replacement therapy. Side-effects can occur and may include anorexia and nausea, postural hypotension, confusional states and delirium. Over a prolonged time, involuntary movements (dyskinesia) and cardiac arrhythmias may develop. Some of these unwanted side-effects can be minimised with the addition of a decarboxylase inhibitor such as carbidopa, which inhibits the conversion of L-dopa into dopamine in organs other than the brain, thereby eliminating those effects due to dopamine in the rest of the body, in particular nausea and vomiting. Both these drugs can be obtained in a variety of combined preparations, e.g. Sinemet, available in two strengths — Sinemet 110, which contains 100 mg of L-dopa and 10 mg of carbidopa, and Sinemet 275, which contains 250 mg of L-dopa and 25 mg of carbidopa. The doses need to be adjusted carefully to suit each person.

Other drugs which may be used, although not nearly so often now, are those of the anticholinergic group. These drugs act by blocking the cholinergic effects which oppose the action of dopamine in the striatum. They include benzhexol (Artane), benztropine (Cogentin) and orphenidrine (Disipal). Side-effects can include dryness of the mouth, constipation and urinary retention, confusion and nocturnal hallucinations. These drugs are sometimes given in the early stages of the disease, L-dopa being reserved for later use.

Mention should be made of amantadine (Symmetrel), an antiviral agent which may be given in doses of 100–400 mg daily, which relieves rigidity and hypokinesia. Why it works is uncertain. Bromocriptine (Parlodel) belongs to a group of drugs that stimulate the post-synaptic dopamine receptors, and is given in a dose of 2.5 mg daily, increasing to 40 mg daily as tolerated. It does, however, produce nausea, dyskinesia and potentially intolerable psychiatric disturbances for the patient.

Surgical treatment involving the creation of lesions in the thalamus is now seldom performed, as the outcome is not always of benefit to the patient, and the outstanding progress made in drug therapy has reduced the number of operations being performed.

Related nursing skills

These patients have a chronic progressive disease. The process is steadily downhill over a number of years, and eventually the patient may become bedridden, requiring full nursing care. It should be added that sensation is retained in Parkinson's disease, and therefore bedsores and bad posturing of limbs will be painful as well as deform the patient. At this advanced stage the mental state of the patient may have deteriorated.

Before this helpless period is reached, the patient may encounter certain problems, not least of all the difficulty of being socially accepted because of his bradykinesia and dysarthria. The nurse who is able to appreciate that his physical slowness does not indicate a corresponding mental inertia should encourage the patient by giving him time to be as independent as possible, and by making an effort to have a conversation despite its difficulties.

This possible social barrier is not helped by the patient's own inhibitions about his tremor, which worsen in times of stress. The feeling of being apart from society often makes him depressed and inclined to stagnate. These factors increase the problems of caring for the patient, who becomes over-critical and very difficult to please; mental and physical activity must be encouraged.

With foresight, patience and a positive approach, the nurse can enhance the patient's self-confidence as well as his independence. The provision of a low bed with a firm base, a comfortable mattress and near the lavatory, eases difficulties of getting in and out of bed, lessens pain in the back (a frequent complaint), and allows for the patient's reduced bladder control and speed (trousers should be zipped and not buttoned). Velcro, a material used to fasten clothing in place of buttons and zips, is another practical aid and may allow the patient to dress himself without help. The patient should sit in a high, winged chair with an upright back and arms, which he will find more supportive and easier to rise from than a low, reclining seat. Once standing, the patient may not be able to walk, and to initiate this the nurse should gently rock him backwards and forwards. Sometimes a patient freezes in a doorway or between items of furniture and is unable to advance; imagining there is a step to get over often helps him to recommence walking. When in bed, the patient will need to be turned if he cannot roll over on his own. At meal times the nurse's help may be required in cutting up food because the patient cannot apply sufficient pressure to the cutlery. Nursing care may also include helping the patient to find suitable stimulants to encourage regular bowel activity.

Many patients can be nursed at home with the support of the community nursing and social services. Special equipment, which the patient has access to in hospital, can be fitted in the home, e.g. safety rails in the bathroom and bedside stairways, a firm mattress on the patient's bed to assist turning, and special cutlery. Some communities may even have a visiting occupational health and physiotherapy service. Simple measures, such as drinking with a bendable straw when the tremor is severe, can be instituted by the patient himself. Anyone suffering from Parkinson's disease should report to the Driving Vehicle Licensing Centre, which may insist on some driving restrictions.

Useful help, and support for sufferers and their relatives with problems that can arise, can be obtained from the Parkinson's Disease Society, which was established in 1969 and now has more than 100 local branches throughout the UK. In a recent survey conducted by the society, it was noted that information about the organisation was only given to 12% of their membership by either a doctor or hospital worker, whereas a far greater number of sufferers found out about the society via newspaper articles and the recommendation of friends. The implications of these results must be clear.

THE SHY–DRAGER SYNDROME

When signs and symptoms of parkinsonism occur in combination with orthostatic hypotension, this is termed the Shy–Drager syndrome. The cause is unknown, and it occurs more often in males between the ages of 50 and 75. The severe hypotension makes it almost impossible for the patient to stand without fainting. Treatment is very difficult; fludrocortisone (Florinef) 0.1–0.6 mg daily may be of some use. Elastic stockings or a space suit may help to reduce the pooling of blood in the legs. Life expectancy is only 7–15 years from onset.

FURTHER READING

ASHWORTH, B. & SAUNDERS, M. (1977) *Management of Neurological Disorders*, p. 81. London: Pitman Medical.

DAVIDSON, D.L.W. & LENMAN, J.A.R. (1981) *Neurological Therapeutics,* p. 73. London: Pitman Medical.

FRANKLIN, S., PERRY, A. & BEATTIE, A. (1982) *Living with Parkinson's Disease.* London: Parkinson's Disease Society.

GRESH, C. (1980) Helpful tips you can give your patients with Parkinson's disease. *Nursing (US), 10*:1, 26.

IVESON-IVESON, J. (1981) Parkinson's disease. *Nursing Mirror, 153*:2, 36.

LEATHERBARROW, L. (1982) In need of support (Parkinson's disease). *Nursing Mirror 154*:2, 44.

LEGG, N.J. (1983) Parkinson's disease: course and management. *The Practitioner, 227*:1377, 375.

OXTOBY, M. (1980) *Parkinson's Disease Patients and Their Social Needs.* London: Parkinson's Disease Society.

WHITELY, A. (1981) We called him Paddington (Parkinson's disease). *Nursing Mirror, 153*:25, 44.

USEFUL ADDRESS

Parkinson's Disease Society
36 Portland Place
London W1N 3DG

17 Disorders of voluntary movement

CENTRAL NERVOUS SYSTEM DISEASE

PARALYSIS

Paralysis (or plegia) denotes loss of power which implies that there would be no response to a painful stimulus. Incomplete loss of power is termed paresis, and can be mild or severe depending on the extent of the damage to the nerves. There is a varying degree of response to a painful stimulus. The area affected is referred to by a prefix, e.g. monoplegia, paralysis of one limb, or hemiparesis, weakness of one half of the body, i.e. arm and leg on the same side and often the face. There are many causes of paralysis and these will be considered briefly.

Hemiplegia

Hemiplegia results from damage to the upper motor neurone in the cerebral hemisphere, and the degree of weakness depends on the extent of the lesion.

Causes

The causes of hemiplegia are:

a. cerebral vascular accident (stroke), e.g. thrombosis of a major artery or haemorrhage into the brain (especially in hypertension);
b. cerebral tumour;
c. head injury;
d. birth injury to the brain, which can result in a congenital hemiparesis and, where both cerebral hemispheres are affected, a double hemiplegia is produced (cerebral diplegia). The weak limbs grow less than normal so that both bones and muscles are smaller.

Clinical features

Tone is increased in the flexors of the upper limb and the extensors of the lower limb so that a characteristic posture results. The arm is held into the body and the elbow, wrist and fingers are flexed. The knee is straight and the foot pointed downwards. As the patient walks, he swings his stiff leg in a half circle to avoid scraping his toes. The clasp-knee phenomenon, where resistance to passive movement is increased and then suddenly yields, is present. At the onset of a cerebral vascular accident, tone of the paralysed limbs is often markedly diminished before the characteristic spasticity develops. Bladder function is not usually disturbed. If the lesion extends into the parietal lobe, there may be loss of sensation in the paralysed limbs and the patient may ignore or even deny that they are defective. In lesions of the dominant hemisphere (usually left) disturbances of speech are prominent.

Paraplegia

Paraplegia results from spinal cord damage, and again the degree of weakness depends on the extent of the lesion.

Causes

The causes of paraplegia are as follows.

1. Trauma, e.g. spinal fracture dislocation.
2. Compression by:
   a. tumour
   (i) in the vertebrae, usually secondary carcinoma from a primary in the breast or lung,
   (ii) inside the meninges,
   (iii) inside the spinal cord,
   b. abscess
   c. cervical or thoracic intervertebral disc prolapse and cervical spondylosis.
3. Ischaemia, e.g. from spinal artery thrombosis.
4. Demyelinating disease, e.g. multiple sclerosis.
5. Degenerative disorders, e.g. motor neurone disease (without sensory loss).

Clinical features

There is loss of sensory and motor function below the level of the lesion. Bladder disturbances are very common, and the patient may have urgency of micturition with incontinence or urinary retention. The tone in the legs is increased, except in sudden onset of paraplegia where an initial flaccid paralysis precedes spasticity. Reflexes are exaggerated and plantar responses extensor.

Flexor spasm

Measures to reduce painful flexor spasm are summarised under 'Related nursing skills'; however, the following medical intervention can also be used in conjunction with physiotherapy and good nursing care.

Medical care

Systemic drugs in use include:

diazepam (Valium) 5–30 mg in daily divided doses;
baclofen (Lioresal) 15–60 mg in daily divided doses;
dantrolene (Dantrium) 50–400 mg in daily divided doses;
chlordiazepoxide (Librium) 30–60 mg in daily divided doses.

These drugs, with the exception of dantrolene, act at spinal level to smooth out muscular activity. Dantrolene acts peripherally, blocking muscular contractions beyond the neuromuscular junction to produce a reduction in spasticity. Unfortunately a major disadvantage in drug treatment is the unwanted side-effects that can produce drowsiness, nausea, psychiatric symptoms and a severe reduction in muscle tone resulting in flaccid limbs upon which the patient cannot weight bear.

Intrathecal drugs. An injection of phenol will damage the nerve roots, causing a lower motor neurone lesion and permanent reduction of spasticity. It also destroys bladder and bowel control, and very careful consideration must be given before using this method.

Perineural injection. Phenol is injected into the appropriate peripheral nerve via a spinal needle. The advantage of this method is that bladder function remains unaffected.

Tenotomy. Division of the tendon of a spastic muscle will relieve the spasm and is occasionally performed when other measures have failed.

Related nursing skills

Those patients who remain permanently paralysed to varying degrees need to depend on skilled nursing care as the mainstay of not only their treatment but also their life. A well-planned care plan will increase the quality and expectancy of each patient's life.

The ease with which patients accept being partially dependent on other people varies greatly. It is important to let each patient do the maximum he can. An encouraging, cheerful attitude will do much to inspire the patient to help himself. The situation is particularly difficult when parietal lobe involvement causes the patient to ignore his paralysed limbs.

Patients with chronic diseases will develop a routine to suit their home circumstances. Hospitalisation of these patients is advisable if complications, e.g. pressure sores or bladder infection, are not resolving. Not only can the patient receive constant medical and nursing care, but the family can have a rest from their exacting duties. Liaison between hospital and community staff gives the patient and his family continuity of care. Most patients can be accommodated successfully in their homes, provided they and their families are given adequate support and encouragement. Regular home visits from the general practitioner, community nurse and social worker are essential.

Under the provision of the Chronic Sick and Disabled Persons Act, home conversions can be undertaken, e.g. widening doors to accommodate a wheelchair and the installation of various bath and toilet aids. Financial assistance is available through the payment of certain allowances, either to the patient or his family. These include invalidity benefit with additional supplements for dependent family members, a mobility allowance, free prescriptions, dental treatment and school meals, an attendance allowance and rent and rates rebates. Certain criteria need to be fulfilled for the allowances, and each patient will be assessed individually to determine which allowances, if any, are payable.

Permanent hospitalisation is avoided for as long as possible, but may become necessary if home conditions cannot be made suitable, e.g. the family reject the patient or, as is more likely, find it impossible to continue as he becomes more disabled. Hospitalisation should, in the case of a young person, be in a Young Chronic Sick Unit and not a geriatric ward.

Positioning the patient

Careful consideration must be given to positioning the paralysed patient in bed, in order to avoid three of the main complications, i.e. contractures, muscle spasm and pressure sores. The patient can be placed in any one of four positions, right and left lateral, prone and supine provided he feels comfortable and there is no other contraindication (Fig. 17.1). Any paralysed limbs must be supported in good alignment. The ankles and feet are dorsiflexed, and the hips and knees are separated and flexed with a pillow. The nonparalysed arm is placed in a comfortable position to suit the patient, and the paralysed arm is maintained in flexion with a suitable object, e.g. a rolled bandage or rubber ball to act as a hand grip.

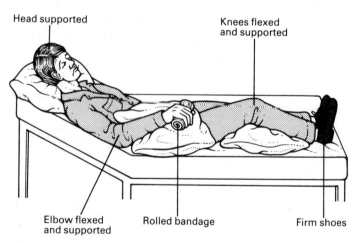

Head supported   Knees flexed and supported

Elbow flexed and supported   Rolled bandage   Firm shoes

Fig. 17.1. *Position for paralysed patient.*

Skin care

The skin is the body's external protective agent, and maintaining this barrier in good condition requires extra attention in patients who are unable to move freely. A bed or immersion bath, with careful attention to the patient's personal hygiene, is performed daily. If he is able to, allow the patient to brush his teeth, comb his hair and shave, or (if a woman) to apply her cosmetics. The patient's finger- and toenails should be trimmed regularly (a chiropodist may be needed if the feet are in poor condition), and his hair washed as necessary. Female patients usually appreciate the services of a hairdresser. Following a patient's bath is often a good time to dress him in his clothes. The patient's skin should be inspected frequently for any breakdown. Pressure sores, once they occur, can be difficult to heal, debilitate the patient and slow down his progress.

Prevention of pressure sore formation receives high priority in the care plan. Tissue death occurs as a result of destruction of the microcirculation to the skin; this can occur when pressures of 30 mmHg or more are inflicted over a period of time on an area of skin (Fig. 17.2). To avoid this complication, the patient will require a

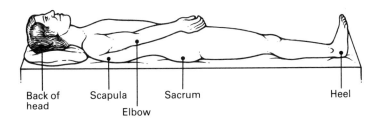

Back of head   Scapula   Elbow   Sacrum   Heel

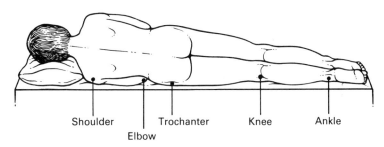

Shoulder   Elbow   Trochanter   Knee   Ankle

Fig. 17.2. *Danger pressure zones.*

regular turning schedule to be organised. Regular repositioning of the patient's body alters the area receiving pressure. Most centres advocate regular 2-hourly turning; however, an alternative system has been devised. This incorporates the use of a turning chart which is based on a 24-hour clock. Various periods of the day are allocated to different positions, and each chart can be altered to suit each patient's individual requirements, i.e. whether the patient is at a high risk or diminished risk of developing pressure necrosis. Several rules need to be borne in mind when devising a schedule.

1. The patient should be nursed flat to achieve better weight distribution, noting that greater pressures are inflicted in the lateral position as opposed to supine or prone.
2. Any time that an area of skin remains under pressure, a corresponding length of time is required to allow the skin to recover.
3. The total maximum length of time within a 24-hour cycle that a patient should be in each of the positions is: supine 8–12 hours, right lateral 5–7 hours, prone 0–8 hours, left lateral 5–7 hours.
4. The turning schedule needs to be modified to allow for any change in the patient's condition.

Other predisposing factors in the development of pressure sores may include: a deviation from the ideal weight, elevation in body temperature, incontinence of urine and faeces, anaemia, poor nutrition, poor lifting techniques, and mismanagement of pressure-relieving aids. If any of these problems arise, appropriate action will need to be taken to correct them. It can be seen from the above that the development of a sore is not an indication of nursing failure.

Redness and chafing indicate that an area is receiving too much pressure, and, if these warnings are unheeded, the skin will break down.

Decubitus ulcer

When a pressure sore develops, the patient must be nursed off the area and have his skin care and pressure-relieving aids reviewed. There are two main types of pressure sore; superficial, in which excoriation of the skin develops and then progresses inwards, and deep sores, which occur within the tissue and spread outwards. The skin areas most prone to breakdown are those in weight-bearing positions over bony prominences. Pressure does not occur only in bed; a patient sitting in a chair can exert a pressure of around 200 mmHg on his sacrum (microcirculation damage occurs at 30 mmHg).

A treatment plan should be drawn up in conjunction with the medical staff, the principles of which should cover:

a. removing the primary cause (i.e. pressure) and correcting any secondary problems (e.g. poor nutrition);
b. cleaning the broken area;
c. debriding any dead tissue (where applicable);
d. providing a therapeutic environment to allow new tissue to granulate.

Removing the primary cause involves reviewing the turning schedule so that all pressure is removed from the compromised area. It may also be necessary to reconsider what pressure-relieving aids are in use and modify them. The sore is measured at two points in order to determine the progress of the necrosis. A suitable cleansing agent will need to be selected, and this will probably depend on local policy. Suitable solutions include povidine-iodine, cetrimide, and hydrogen peroxide. When there is dead tissue present, this will need to be removed as its presence will impede growth of any new tissue. The easiest way to remove slough is with an enzymatic debriding agent, e.g. Aserbine cream or lotion. Surgical removal may be considered where there is a large area of tissue involved; this would be followed by plastic surgery to create a new skin flap.

A clean therapeutic environment is now required to complete the healing process. In recent years many new products have appeared which all claim to be the answer; however, this does not appear to be the case. A bewildering choice faces the nurse and the use of some of the products will be determined by local policy, and in some cases cost. Examples include the following.

1. Debrisan: dry porous beads are placed on the sore and secretions from the wound are drawn into their interspaces. The beads absorb the fluid and swell, providing a moist medium and protective layer below which epithelialisation can occur.
2. The application of a thin self-adhesive, transparent film which

is waterproof, non-porous but permeable to air and water will also provide an appropriate environment to encourage epithelialisation. An example of such a product is Op-site.

Both these new products are fairly costly, and there are many traditional and cheaper methods, e.g. the application of a sugar paste to a sore is said to be beneficial, and placing karaya-gum rings around the margins of a sore with karaya powder on the sore itself has also been found to be of use.

Whichever method is chosen, an aseptic technique is required during every procedure.

Several myths have developed around treating and preventing pressure sores, and in many cases there is now scientific evidence to refute them. These include the use of alcohol as a 'rub' and the application of dry oxygen blowing over a sore; even massage comes in for criticism (it has been demonstrated that, when performed too vigorously, massage actually destroys the vital microcirculation).

Pressure-relieving aids

Many pressure-relieving aids are now available, and only a few are mentioned here. They can be used both prophylactically and in the treatment of sores. There are three main types of aids: those which minimise pressure, those which assist in turning patients, and those designed to support specific areas.

Ripple beds are electrically operated, air-filled plastic mattresses divided into horizontal bands 5–10 cm wide. Alternate bands fill with air and then deflate, giving a very slow rippling effect. This alters the areas subjected to pressure. The pump is adjusted so that a comfortable supportive mattress is provided. A water bed is another example of a device that can be used to minimise pressure.

The second category of pressure-relieving aids includes those aids which assist in turning the patient, and examples of these include the Stryker–Circoelectric bed and the Egerton Net suspension bed. These beds are designed to allow the nurse to turn the patient more frequently and with the minimum of staff and effort. Aids such as sheepskins and gel pads can be used to support specific areas, such as the heels.

Diet

The dietary intake of a paralysed patient can, for most, be normal. A high roughage diet may be indicated in those patients experiencing problems with bowel motions, and a soft diet in those with swallowing difficulties. The patient is encouraged to feed himself, and the occupational therapist can provide specially adapted cutlery and crockery to assist him in this task. Patients with sensory impairment will need to use an insulated beaker for hot drinks.

Bowels

Retraining of the bowel will be required, the aim of which is to produce a formed movement at regular intervals. A high roughage diet and regular laxatives are used. Occasionally an enema or manual evacuation will be required, and this needs to be attended to with the minimum of fuss as the patient will feel quite embarrassed and upset at this distasteful procedure.

Bladder

Initially an indwelling catheter will be used; however, it is desirable to remove it and replace it with an alternative device, such as a re-usable condom appliance which diverts the urine into a leg bag. This device can only be used in men; at the moment there is no equivalent device for women.

Ideally, retraining the bladder is probably the most satisfying and acceptable alternative for the patient. This involves determining whether or not the bladder is atonic; if it is, manual expression at regular intervals and at specific times of the day is needed and if there is still a reflex tone, determining trigger spots and then stimulating them to induce a urinary flow are required. Both methods are difficult to master and a great deal of patience is required by both the patient and the nurse if the outcome is to be successful.

A daily fluid intake of 2000 ml is needed in order to prevent the formation of calculi and urinary tract infection.

Flexor spasm

When spastic paraplegia is marked, painful flexor spasm may occur.

These involuntary movements of the hips and knees limit mobility, and sitting may become impossible. Good positioning (as previously discussed) will assist greatly in reducing spasm. A programme of passive range of movement exercises is drawn up and performed by the nurse and the physiotherapist, the aims of which are to preserve mobility of the joints, to reduce spasticity and spasm, and to maintain good circulation by stimulation of the muscles. The application of cold ice packs may produce temporary relief, although this is only performed under very close supervision. The use of drugs and tenotomy is discussed under medical care.

Occupational therapy

The paralysed patient will benefit from tasks selected to improve muscle power, co-ordination and range of movements in joints. Activities include remedial games such as draughts, in which grips and weights of the playing pieces are adapted to suit the patient. Bimanual occupations such as sanding, sawing or polishing can be assisted by slings and springs. The patient's morale must be maintained and his achievements constantly emphasised. Not only does he require considerable help in coping with the activities of daily living, but he may need to be guided into new hobbies and interests before old pastimes become impossible.

The possum

See p. 162.

Mobility

The patient is encouraged to gain his independence through mobility. This may involve learning to walk again with the use of a walking stick or zimmer or leg calipers. Once again, the advice of the physiotherapist should be sought. Some patients will only become mobile through the use of a wheelchair, and it is important that the correct model is selected. In some instances an electrically driven wheelchair is indicated.

Discharge

Some patients will eventually be discharged home after what has been a very long time spent in hospital care. The process is a slow one, with the patient going home for a few hours only on the first day and then returning to the hospital at night. As the patient and his family become more confident, the length of time spent at home can be gradually increased.

It is important that each member of the family knows what is involved in caring for the patient and what his daily needs will be. Liaison with the community staff is vital; nurses, social workers and the patient's general practitioner all need to be involved in the patient's care, and ideally the community nurse should visit the patient in hospital prior to discharge so that a rapport can be developed. A visit to the patient's home is also desirable so that any major problems can be averted, making the patient's discharge a smoother process.

ATAXIA

Ataxia is a loss of co-ordination of movement so that a smooth, direct action becomes irregular and inaccurate. This may be due to the following.

Sensory disturbance

Inadequate information from muscles and joints on the range and speed of movements performed results in inco-ordination of further movements. The sensory loss may be due to peripheral neuropathy or spinal cord disorders involving the posterior columns, e.g. tabes dorsalis, multiple sclerosis and subacute combined degeneration of the cord.

Cerebellar disturbance

If a lesion, e.g. a tumour or infarction, involves one-half of the cerebellum, then ataxia occurs in the limbs on the same side of the body. Irregularity of rate, range, direction and force of movement may be demonstrated by the finger–nose–finger test or the heel–knee–shin test. An intention tremor is also frequently seen. A midline lesion of the cerebellum causes the trunk to become ataxic, and sitting, standing and walking are all unsteady and broad based. Nystagmus, which is most marked on the side of the lesion, commonly occurs, and inco-ordination of speech produces dysarthria of the scanning speech type.

The common diseases affecting the cerebellum are multiple sclerosis and tumour, i.e. medulloblastoma in children and haemangioblastoma and metastases in adults. Some drugs, e.g. phenytoin and alcohol, cause reversible cerebellar dysfunction.

Rare degenerative disorders that involve the cerebellum are due to hypothyroidism, distant carcinoma (usually of the ovary or bronchus) and certain hereditary disorders, of which Friedreich's ataxia is the most frequently encountered.

Friedreich's ataxia

In Friedreich's ataxia, which can effect either sex, there is degeneration of the spinal cord as well as of the cerebellum. The resultant weakness and ataxia cause progressive difficulty in walking, and this becomes apparent before the child is 10 years old. The feet have high arches (pes cavus) and scoliosis of the spine is often present. Sensory disturbances, depressed tendon reflexes and extensor plantar responses develop, and sometimes nystagmus and scanning speech are features. No treatment can halt the progression of the disease, which eventually confines the patient to a wheelchair.

Nursing care is similar to that required for patients chronically disabled with muscular dystrophy or multiple sclerosis. Death usually occurs in the second or third decade as a result of the cardiomyopathy which is associated with this condition.

Related nursing skills

Even though there may be no weakness, ataxia alone can cause a severe disability, and in a mentally alert patient considerable frustration occurs. The intention tremor becomes worse on voluntary movement and this leads to difficulty in feeding, writing and walking. The nurse must be observant and helpful if accidents, such as burns from spilt hot drinks and injuries from falling or bumping into furniture and doorposts, are to be avoided. Certain aids, e.g. walking frames, bendable straws, non-slip mats, clip-on plate rims and specially adapted cutlery, reduce the risk of accidents and increase independence. The latter consideration is very important to most patients.

PERIPHERAL NEUROMUSCULAR SYSTEM DISEASE

Muscle weakness may be due to disease of the muscle fibres or of its nerve supply.

MUSCLE FIBRE DISEASE

Muscle fibre disease may be a hereditary disorder (muscular dystrophy), an inflammatory process (myositis), or associated with a metabolic disorder.

The cause of muscular dystrophy remains unknown, and several theories have been postulated.

1. The myopathic theory, in which there is thought to be a biochemical abnormality within the muscle itself.
2. The neurovascular theory, in which the capillary circulation to the muscle is thought to be defective.
3. The neurogenic theory, in which motor units within the anterior horn are thought to be destroyed or immobilised.
4. The membrane theory, in which there is thought to be a disorder of the cell membrane of the muscles and other tissues.

Muscular dystrophies (myopathies)

Pseudohypertrophic muscular dystrophy (Duchenne disease). Pseudohypertrophic muscular dystrophy is inherited as a sex-linked recessive character. It therefore affects boys, whereas their sisters may, like their mothers, carry the abnormal gene and pass it to their sons.

Duchenne muscular dystrophy is by far the most common, and unfortunately the most devastating.

The diagnosis is made between the ages of 3 and 5 years, and the signs of the disease begin with wasting and weakness of the calf and shoulder muscles, which are initially belied by deposits of fat that add to their bulk. Then the hip muscles are affected and the child develops a waddling gait. He falls easily and then has difficulty

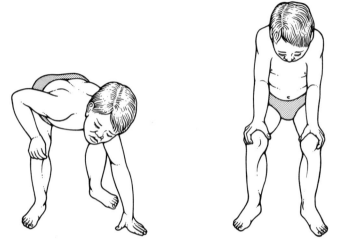

Fig. 17.3. *'Climbing up legs' to demonstrate how a child with muscular dystrophy rises from the floor.*

rising, but learns to push himself upright by climbing up his own legs (Fig. 17.3). Weakness of the trunk muscles leads to scoliosis. There is no sensory disturbance.

The progressive wasting of muscles with accompanying weakness continues until walking is impossible and the patient is wheelchair bound or bedridden. Patients usually succumb to a chest infection before the age of 15 years.

Benign X-linked Becker dystrophy. Onset does not usually occur until the child is at least 5 years old, and the disorder may not manifest itself until the early twenties. A history of weakness similar to that found in Duchenne dystrophy is encountered, and the differential diagnosis is made on the later onset and less rapid progression of the disease.

Limb-girdle dystrophy. Limb-girdle dystrophy can occur in both sexes and it is of autosomal recessive inheritance, and affects, as the name implies, the shoulder or pelvic-girdle muscles. Onset is usually between the ages of 20 and 35 years. Progression of the disability can be variable; some patients may remain unaffected for the next 20 years of their life, whereas others will develop a degree of weakness.

Facioscapulo-humeral dystrophy. This type of dystrophy typically affects the muscles of the face and shoulders first, and is diagnosed in late adolescence. It affects both sexes equally and is a relatively mild form of the disorder. Progress of the symptoms, which is usually very slow, is noted when the lower limbs become affected, resulting in bilateral footdrop.

Investigations

The enzyme creatine phosphokinase is released into the blood as the muscles degenerate, and very high levels are apparent in the early stages of the disease. Electromyogram studies demonstrate myopathic changes, and muscle biopsy shows atrophy of the muscle fibres.

Fortunately, although she has no clinical evidence of myopathy, a woman carrying the abnormal gene can be identified by the finding of a moderately raised serum creatine phosphokinase level. Having been warned, she may decide to have no children; however, because it is now possible to determine the sex of the child in early pregnancy, she may use this service and opt for an abortion if the fetus is male.

Treatment

There is no treatment which influences the course of this disease, and care is directed at making the child's life as tolerable as possible. About half of the children have some intellectual impairment as well as their increasing physical disability, and special schooling is usually required.

As the weakness progresses, the child relies first on crutches and then on a wheelchair to maintain his mobility. Leg irons and toe-raising devices may prove useful. Physiotherapy to prevent contractures, and nursing care to avoid pressure sores become important as the disease advances. Any respiratory infection must be treated promptly (often in hospital) with antibiotics and intensive physiotherapy because the weakness of the chest muscles prevents adequate coughing.

Related nursing skills

Duchenne-type dystrophy is the most devastating, and therefore provides the nurse with the most problems. Many children will be managed within the community, provided that the home circumstances are reasonably good and that effective support is provided by community personnel, the most important of whom will be the nurse and/or health visitor.

The parents, who have often seen an elder son or uncle die of the disease, require sympathetic support and tuition in practical nursing in order to provide for their invalid son. Pressure sores, contractures and chest or urinary tract infections are the main problems, and the parents will need to know about these and how to minimise them.

If a major complication occurs or if the disease advances to a degree where the child cannot be managed at home, admission to hospital is necessary. The Social Work Department will be able to provide addresses of organisations which provide holidays for muscular dystrophy sufferers, which will permit the parents to have a break on their own. An example of such an organisation is the Muscular Dystrophy Group of Great Britain, which also provides a welfare, education and information service for sufferers and their families.

Financial support can be provided: the parents may qualify for an attendance allowance, and adaptations to the home can be arranged through the Social Work Department. As the child grows older, he or she may qualify for invalidity benefit, if unable to work, and also a mobility allowance.

Education

In the Duchenne-type dystrophy, there is often intellectual impairment requiring attendance at a special school with teachers who are trained and experienced in these kinds of problems. It has been suggested that attendance at a normal school where possible will be of far greater benefit for the wheelchair bound child. It allows the child to live in a normal environment and permits the other children to realise that a disabled person is still a person, except that he has some special problems. This can only be undertaken in very special circumstances.

Genetic counselling

When the diagnosis of muscular dystrophy has been confirmed, particularly in the Duchenne type, then investigations should be performed on the mother and any other closely connected females within the family.

Elevated creatine phosphokinase levels are found in 80% of carriers, and each individual should be informed of the outcome of her test. Depending on probability, the female may be advised not to have any children; however, this information can only be provided by a genetic counsellor.

Dystrophy myotonica

Dystrophy myotonica is a hereditary disorder which affects either sex. It becomes apparent in early adulthood and slowly progresses over the following 40–50 years. One rare version, myotonia congenita, occurs in childhood. The wasting and weakness begin in the hips and shoulders (limb girdles) and the facial muscles. The patient develops a markedly scrawny neck which, when combined with ptosis and (in men) frontal baldness, produces a characteristic appearance. Other features include cataract, testicular atrophy, and a curious mental attitude in which the patient denies the disease process.

Myotonia, i.e. continued contraction of a muscle beyond the required length of time, may be demonstrated by shaking hands with the patient, who has difficulty in relaxing his grip, and by firmly tapping an atrophied muscle, which will become indented because the contraction is maintained.

Treatment

Although there is no treatment which halts the very slow progression of weakness, procainamide (Pronestyl) 250 mg four times daily, phenytoin (Epanutin) 100 mg three times daily, or quinine 300 mg daily, all reduce the myotonia. If the neck muscles become very weak, a collar may be needed to support the head, and when the chest muscles are affected, respiratory infections must be treated in hospital.

The other muscular dystrophies are much less common and have varying modes of inheritance, ages of onset, and speeds of progression. They normally take their names from the muscles predominantly affected, e.g. ocular myopathy.

Related nursing skills are similar to those for muscular dystrophy.

Inflammatory disorders of muscles (myositis)

Inflammation may be confined to one group of muscles (myositis) or generalised (polymyositis), and sometimes there is an overlying skin rash (dermatomyositis). The affected muscles are very tender and the patient is febrile.

The cause of the inflammation is usually a collagen disease, e.g. systemic lupus erythematosus or polyarteritis nodosa, but it may result from a serum sickness-type reaction or hidden carcinoma.

On investigation, the serum creatine phosphokinase level is raised because of the muscle damage, and the erythrocyte sedimentation rate (ESR) is often very high because of the inflammation. Other investigations include tests to find the underlying disorder, e.g. examination of the blood for evidence of collagen disease, and chest x-ray, barium meal and enema to exclude a carcinoma. Muscle biopsy shows the inflammatory process and the blood vessels may exhibit changes of polyarteritis nodosa.

Treatment

Steroids remain the mainstay of treatment; prednisolone (Prednesol) 60 mg per day is given and then gradually reduced over 6 months as the symptoms subside. In some patients a dose of 5–20 mg daily of prednisolone may be required indefinitely. Patients with a rapid onset and early diagnosis respond best to treatment, whereas patients with an underlying carcinoma do not do as well. Immunosuppressive drugs have recently been used in those patients who do not respond to steroid therapy. Azathioprine (Imuran) 50–300 mg daily and cyclophosphamide (Endoxanal) 100–300 mg daily have both been tried.

Analgesia will be required during the acute inflammatory stage, and complete bedrest will also be necessary. Once the pain has been controlled, passive range of movement exercises may be introduced by the physiotherapist, although this mode of treatment has been questioned.

A more chronic form of polymyositis, that leads to wasting and weakness with little or no pain, can occur as result of sarcoidosis, but generally the cause is not known. It is diagnosed by electromyogram studies and muscle biopsy. Unfortunately the response to prednisolone is variable.

Related nursing skills. Complete bedrest is essential, as the patient finds that the slightest movement can cause a lot of pain. Measures to avoid the complications of bed rest such as pressure sores, chest infection, or deep venous thrombosis will need to be taken. Anti-embolism stockings and the use of a special bed, e.g. a water bed, for comfort may be indicated. The provision of adequate analgesia prior to performing potentially painful nursing procedures cannot be over-emphasised. Because of the patient's reluctance to move in bed, effective care of the skin will be required, and frequent inspections of all the pressure points should be performed 2-hourly. Any sign of deterioration in the integrity of the skin should be noted and appropriate action taken to avoid further damage.

When steroids are given in such large doses, various side-effects can occur. These may include gastric disturbances, salt and water retention producing peripheral oedema, hypertension and hypokalaemia causing generalised weakness, moon face and osteoporosis. Diabetes may be precipitated or exacerbated. Measures can be taken to counteract some of the side-effects; potassium supplements may be given in accordance with serum electrolyte results. Some sources advocate administering cimetedine (Tagamet) routinely to avoid gastric ulcerations, whereas others may give the medication with a glass of milk, preferably following a meal. Urine should be tested daily for glucose content. Steroids should be decreased gradually, and some centres may employ the use of a steroid-reducing chart.

Metabolic causes of muscle disease

Thyrotoxicosis. The wasting and weakness of the limb girdles and eye muscles, which sometimes develop secondarily to thyrotoxicosis, usually recover when the thyroid disease is treated.

Cushing's syndrome. A proximal myopathy may become apparent in this condition, especially if the disorder is induced by therapeutic steroids; it tends to be resolved if steroids are reduced or withdrawn.

Myxoedema. In severe myxoedema, there may be a myopathy which usually responds to treatment with thyroxin.

Acromegaly. A myopathy can occur due to the excess secretion of ACTH.

Hypothyroidism. Widespread muscle weakness and atrophy can occur, which improve when the hypothyroidism is treated.

Addison's disease. Muscle wasting and weakness can occur (Addison's myopathy).

Electrolyte imbalance. Lack of calcium, sodium and potassium can produce weakness. In addition, some patients have a hereditary tendency to fluctuations in potassium balance which results in episodes of weakness, i.e. familial periodic paralysis.

Hypokalaemic periodic paralysis. This may last only a few hours or several days, and is usually brought on following a period of vigorous exercise. The serum potassium falls and is treated by the administration of potassium supplements.

Hyperkalaemic periodic paralysis. The serum potassium rises to an abnormally high level. It tends to occur in children, with attacks following exercise and lasting 1–3 hours. It seldom requires treatment but, if indicated, calcium gluconate may be given.

Malignant hyperpyrexia

There is no obvious sign of illness until there is exposure to anaesthetic agents, particularly halothane (Fluothane), when the patient develops hyperpyrexia, metabolic acidosis, tachycardia and rigidity. Treatment consists of discontinuing the anaesthesia and actively cooling the patient with the use of ice packs. Drug therapy which may be useful includes sodium bicarbonate to correct the acidosis, and dantrolene (Dantrium) which inhibits muscle contracture. Mannitol and steroids may also be used. The condition is frequently fatal.

Glycogen storage disorders

These are rare disorders which are in most cases untreatable; they include Pompe's disease (acid-maltase deficiency), McArdle's disease (myophosphorylase deficiency), Cori's disease and Tarui's disease.

Muscle pain develops during exertion due to the patient's inability to degrade glycogen. The only treatment is to advise the patient to avoid vigorous exercise, or alternatively to ingest some glucose prior to exercise.

DISEASES OF THE NERVE SUPPLY TO THE MUSCLES

Acute or chronic lesions of the anterior horn cells or the lower motor neurones leads to muscle weakness and, if prolonged, to wasting. The anterior horn cells are affected acutely by anterior poliomyelitis and involved in chronic degeneration in motor neurone disease. Acute disorders of peripheral nerves include Bell's palsy and acute infective polyneuritis, and chronic lesions include pressure palsies and some hereditary forms of peripheral neuropathy, of which peroneal muscular atrophy is the commonest.

Anterior poliomyelitis

This disorder affects the motor cells in the anterior horn of the grey matter, and is caused by the organism enterovirus, which inhabits the intestine. Elaboration of treatment and related nursing skills can be found in Chapter 8.

Motor neurone disease

Motor neurone disease, which is of unknown aetiology, involves degeneration (in varying proportions) of both upper and lower neurones of the spinal cord and bulbar nuclei. It can take several forms:

- *a.* progressive muscular atrophy;
- *b.* amyotrophic lateral sclerosis;
- *c.* progressive bulbar palsy.

It mainly attacks middle-aged males and produces the characteristic features of progressive wasting of muscles (lower motor neurone lesion), with exaggeration of tendon reflexes (upper motor neurone lesion). Fasciculation occurs in the affected muscles. There is no sensory loss or intellectual impairment. Involvement of the bulbar muscles causes unintelligible speech and dysphagia. This may occur early on in the course of the disease or only afflict the patient in the terminal stages. Death, usually from a respiratory infection, occurs about 2 years after the onset of the disease.

Related nursing skills

There is no medical treatment, and the patient is distressingly aware of this as his disability steadily increases. Many patients can be nursed initially within their home environment, provided that adequate support is provided for the family.

Prior to discharge from hospital, enquiries should be made regarding the patient's home background, especially the suitability of the layout of his home in regard to his present disability. It should be established if other members of the family will be available to assist the patient and, if not, community support will need to be provided. It is useful if while in hospital the patient can meet the personnel who will be visiting him at home, as this helps to establish a rapport.

The patient with motor neurone disease will present with many problems, e.g. physical hygiene, excretion, skin care, general mobility, all of which have been discussed in detail in Chapters 15, 16 and earlier in this. However, two major problems which require important mention are communication and nutrition.

The weakness of the muscles of the face make the patient's speech very difficult to understand, and this will unfortunately deteriorate to indistinguishable noises only. Despite the obvious difficulties, a means of communication needs to be developed so that a total dissociation from the world does not occur. There are few conditions that upset a mentally alert patient more than being unable to make himself understood. It is helpful to elicit as much information as possible early on in the disease, while the patient can communicate reasonably well, which will help to enhance nursing care in the future. Brief, regular conversations are more beneficial and the patient should be given plenty of time to reply and say what he wants to say despite the temptation to always finish the sentence for him. The advice of a speech therapist should be obtained. As the disease progresses, communication may be reduced to blinking 'Yes' and 'No' answers. Where possible, the use of an electric typewriter attached to a possum machine may be a suitable alternative for the patient.

When dysphagia becomes apparent, the patient will appreciate having his food cut up into small pieces, and also the use of specially built up cutlery. Because eating the meal may take a long time, a means of keeping the food hot is essential. For an adult to be fed is a humiliating experience, therefore special arrangements may be required to allow the patient to continue feeding himself for as long as possible. This may be messy and embarrassing for the patient, therefore he should be given privacy without overlooking the social value of mealtimes. Eventually a soft diet is necessary to avoid choking, and from that a liquidised diet given via a nasogastric tube is the next step.

Difficulty in swallowing saliva leads to constant dribbling, which may be reduced with the administration of atropine sulphate 0.6 mg twice daily. When the patient is lying down, a soft paper handkerchief placed under the side of the face will collect any saliva.

Bell's palsy

Bell's palsy is a lower motor neurone paralysis of the facial nerve, the aetiology of which is unknown. The patient exhibits sudden, complete flaccid paralysis of the affected half of his face and his inability to close his eye may necessitate the performance of a tarsorrhaphy, which involves stitching the eyelids together to protect the cornea. Dribbling and difficulty in keeping the paralysed side of the mouth clear of solid food are additional problems. The condition usually begins to resolve after 3 or 4 weeks, but recovery is not always complete.

Acute peripheral neuritis

The commonest cause of acute peripheral neuritis is the Guillain–Barré syndrome, also called acute infective polyneuritis (inflammation of many nerves). This condition is probably not a true infection of the nerves, but an allergic response to a viral infection during the previous 1 to 2 weeks, usually an upper respiratory tract illness with sore throat and malaise. Further information can be found in Chapter 8.

Pressure palsies

Pressure palsies are described in full in Chapter 19.

Peroneal muscular atrophy (Charcot–Marie–Tooth disease)

This develops during adolescence or early adult life, and can affect either sex. Initially the muscles of the foot and then the lower leg become wasted, with a resultant bilateral footdrop, forcing the patient to adopt a high-stepping gait. The muscle wasting is characteristic in that it suddenly halts halfway up the affected limb, producing an inverted bottle appearance.

The feet and hands are usually blue and cold, and there may be some glove-and-stocking sensory loss. When the footdrop is severe, the patient may benefit from special supports.

The wasting process is slowly progressive, but life is not usually shortened. Diagnosis is made from nerve conduction studies and a family history of similar disease.

FURTHER READING

Central nervous system

DAVIS, B. (1982) Claiming benefits—1, Attendance allowance. *Nursing Times, 78*:12, 504.

DAVIS, B. (1982) Claiming benefits—2, Mobility allowance. *Nursing Times 78*:13, 527.

DAVIS, B. (1982) Claiming benefits—3, Maternity allowance. *Nursing Times 78*:14, 572.

DAVIS, B. (1982) Claiming benefits—4, Supplementary benefits and heating additions. *Nursing Times, 78*:15, 630.

DAVIS, B. (1982) Claiming allowances—5, Supplementary benefits and cash additions. *Nursing Times, 78*:16, 662.

DAVIS, B. (1982) Claiming benefits—6, Housing benefits, *Nursing Times, 78*:17, 722.

FALLON, B. (1975) So you're paralysed. London: Spinal Injuries Association.

LOWTHIAN, P. (1979) Turning clock system to prevent pressure sores. *Nursing Mirror, 148*:21, 30.

LOWTHIAN, P. (1982) A review of pressure sore pathogenesis. *Nursing Times, 78*:3, 117.

NEWMAN, P. & WEST, J. (1981) Pressure sores—2, The value of the Norton Score. Occasional Papers. *Nursing Times, 77*:21.

NORTON, D. (1975) Research and the problem of pressure sores. *Nursing Mirror, 140*:7, 65.

ROGERS, E.C. (1979) Paralysed patients and their nursing care. *Nursing (UK)*, 1st series, *5*, 207.

ROGERS, M.A. (1978) *Paraplegia — A Handbook of Practical Care and Advice*. London: Faber and Faber.
ROGERS, M.A. (1979) Paralysis— how it affects movement and daily life. *Nursing (UK)*, 1st series, *5*, 203.
SMITH, B. (1983) Points under pressure. *Nursing Mirror, 156*:16, 24.

Peripheral neuromuscular system disease

BROWN, J.C. (1982) Muscular dystrophy. *The Practitioner, 226*:1368, 1031.
CURRIE, S. (1982) Inflammatory myopathies. *The Practitioner, 226*:1368, 1039.
DAVIDSON, D.L.W. & LENMAN, J.A.R. (1982) *Neurological Therapeutics*, p. 224. London: Pitman Medical.
HARPER, P.S. (1982) Myotonic disorders. *The Practitioner, 226*:1368, 1065.
HOSKING, G. (1980) A decrease in mobility. *Nursing Mirror, 150*:10, 24.
HOSKING, G. (1982) Muscular dystrophy. *Health Visitor, 55*:1, 22.
HOSKING, G. (1982) *An Introduction to Paediatric Neurology*, p. 178. London: Faber and Faber.
MacDONALD, R. (1982) A case of getting used to it (peroneal muscular atrophy). *Nursing Mirror, 155*:9, 15.
McKERAN, R.O. (1976) The muscular dystrophies. *Nursing Times, 72*:39, 1515.
ROSE, V. (1982) Motor neurone disease. *Journal of District Nursing, 1*:2, 4.
ROSS, F. (1980) Motor neurone disease. *Nursing Times, 76*:41, 1789.
RUSSELL, P. (1978) *The Wheelchair Child*. Human Horizons Series. London: Souvenir Press.
SUMMERS, D.H. (1981) Motor neurone disease. *Nursing Times*, Occasional Papers. *177*:1.
WILSON, B. (1982) Battling with motor neurone disease. *British Medical Journal, 284*:34.
ZAKARIAN, T. (1981) Malignant hyperpyrexia — a rare anaesthetic hazard. *Nursing Times, 77*:48, 2048.

USEFUL ADDRESSES

Chest, Heart and Stroke Association
Tavistock House North
Tavistock Square
London WC1H 9JE

Muscular Dystrophy Group of Great Britain
Nattrass House
35 McAulay Road
London SW4 0QB

18 Disorders of involuntary movement

Uncontrollable involuntary movements, which may range from a mild tremor to exhausting dramatic actions, can be extremely distressing and socially embarrassing for the patient. Treatment of these disorders is largely unsatisfactory, being limited to drug therapy and psychological support.

TREMOR

Tremor is due to rhythmical alternating contraction and relaxation in antagonistic muscle groups. It may result from fatigue, emotion or disease, and the distribution, rate and rhythm help indicate the cause. Essential tremor is often familial, affecting the hands and being most marked under stress. It appears to diminish if the patient consumes alcohol, but the treatment of choice is propranalol (Inderal) 60–120 mg daily.

Senile tremor

Senile tremor affects the head, lips and hands in the elderly; its character resembles the parkinsonian tremor, but its distribution differs.

Intention tremor

This is described under multiple sclerosis (p. 204). It also occurs in other cerebellar disorders, e.g. degenerations and tumours. Toxins such as excess alcohol, mercury and certain drugs, such as phenytoin, often affect the functioning of the cerebellum and produce tremor. An intention tremor is absent at rest and increases as a voluntary movement is executed. This distinguishes it from a parkinsonian tremor, which is present at rest and reduced on voluntary movement.

Anxiety tremor

A fine tremor seen in some normal people under emotional stress, anxiety tremor is more constantly observed in patients with psychiatric disorders.

Thyrotoxic tremor

This is a fine tremor of outstretched hands, as seen in hyperthyroidism.

Metabolic tremor

Metabolic tremor is a coarse, flapping tremor of the outstretched hands, occurring in advanced stages of hepatic, renal and respiratory failure.

CHOREA

In chorea, there are rapid, jerky involuntary (choreiform) movements of the limbs. They are unrelieved by rest or voluntary action and are associated with involuntary grimacing. The patient may become embarrassed and exhausted by his inability to keep still.

Huntington's chorea

Huntington's chorea is a rare familial disease of the cerebral cortex and basal ganglia. The insidious and progressive onset usually occurs between the ages of 30 and 45 years and is apparent as violent involuntary choreiform movements of the limbs, face and trunk, and progressive dementia leading to bizarre behavioural problems. Mobility becomes affected because of the unstable gait and the patient eventually becomes chair- or bedridden. Communication and feeding problems develop due to dysarthria and dysphagia. The involuntary movements usually disappear when the patient is asleep. Mental deterioration will be seen, in the form of mood swings: the patient will be elated one minute and depressed the next. Irritability and aggression are common features and the patient often neglects his personal appearance and habits. This disorder can affect either sex, and death occurs within 10–15 years, usually from cardiac or respiratory failure due to exhaustion. Inheritance of Huntington's chorea is by a dominant mode and thus half of the children of an affected person will develop the disease. It is tragic that the patient has frequently started a family before realising that he has the condition.

Treatment is difficult; haloperidol (Serenace) or chlorpromazine (Largactil) and tetrabenazine (Nitoman) are the drugs of choice, plus other symptomatic medications such as hypnotics and antidepressants.

Sydenham's chorea (St Vitus' dance)

Mainly a disease of children, although on occasion seen in pregnant women, this chorea is a manifestation of rheumatic fever and is always accompanied by rheumatic carditis. The chorea resolves, although it may last several months, but the cardiac lesions may be fatal. Treatment is similar to that for Huntington's chorea.

Hemiballismus

This, often unilateral, symptom is rare. The violent throwing movements of the arm or leg are usually due to a vascular lesion in the subthalamic nucleus. Treatment is with the use of major tranquillisers.

HEMIFACIAL SPASM

This primarily consists of an irregular twitching of one side of the face. It may follow Bell's palsy.

TICS

Tics are repeated small movements, usually of the eye, which develop as habit spasm in children. They tend to resolve in adulthood, without specific treatment. In some children the tic may be accompanied by abnormal noises such as a bark or squeal — a condition known as the Gilles de la Tourette syndrome.

ATHETOSIS, DYSKINESIA AND DYSTONIA

Athetosis, dyskinesia and dystonia are slow, withering movements involving the limbs, trunk and face. Their treatment is difficult, but in severe cases stereotaxis can sometimes be of benefit.

Athetosis

Athetosis results from jaundice in the neonatal period and is therefore seen in children with rhesus incompatibility.

Facial dyskinesia

Pouting and grimacing may be caused by phenothiazine derivatives. Discontinuing the drug responsible will abate the condition.

Torsion dystonia

There is no obvious cause for the twisting movements of torsion dystonia. A local manifestation is spasmodic torticollis (wry neck), where the neck muscles are affected causing intermittent deviation of the head. This disorder can be treated medically with tranquillisers or surgically by rhizotomy, i.e. division of the spinal nerve roots. Both produce variable results. Torsion dystonia may also involve the limbs or the trunk, producing a more disabling condition, dystonia musculorum deformans.

MYOCLONUS

Myoclonus consists of repeated muscle jerks of the limbs and trunk. It is considered a manifestation of epilepsy, and therefore the administration of an anticonvulsant is the treatment of choice.

TORTICOLLIS

Twisting of the neck occurs as a result of severe muscle spasm and the cause is unknown. Treatment is disappointing, although some patients do recover spontaneously.

WILSON'S DISEASE (HEPATOLENTICULAR DEGENERATION)

Wilson's disease is a familial disorder of metabolism which causes copper to accumulate in the liver and brain and be excreted in the urine. It becomes apparent between the ages of 6 and 20 years and, if untreated, is fatal. The neurological features of rigidity with parkinsonian tremor or wing-beating movements of the arms are accompanied by cirrhosis and hepatic failure. Copper is also deposited in the cornea, where it can be seen as the yellowish-brown Kayser–Fleischer ring under the slit lamp. Treatment is with pencillimine (Cuprimine) 250–500 mg three times daily, the side-effects of which are anorexia, nausea, and diminution or total loss of taste perception. Pyridoxine depletion is corrected with replacement pyridoxine (Benadon). This drug slowly increases the urinary excretion of copper by removing the deposits in the basal ganglia and liver. The patient shows a marked improvement, but maintenance treatment is necessary.

RELATED NURSING SKILLS

The nursing care required for these patients will be determined by the severity of the involuntary movements. Many patients will manage adequately at home by adopting simple preventive measures, e.g. patients with an arm tremor should not handle hot cups of tea. Some patients will learn to avoid those situations which place them under stress and hence exacerbate the tremor.

Patients suffering from Wilson's disease will require a great deal more nursing care. The nursing care plan should incorporate personal hygiene; an alternative means of communication; attention to nutritional needs (a semi-solid, high-protein or low-copper diet may be indicated); an accurate record of fluid balance; careful oral hygiene, particularly in those patients with loss of taste perception; positional changes (incorporating the use of pressure-relieving aids); passive range of movement exercises; chest physiotherapy and occupational therapy.

FURTHER READING

BERK, P.A. (1982) Dyskinesia: nursing care and surgical intervention. *Journal of Neurosurgical Nursing, 14*:1, 23.

DRAPO, P.J. (1981) Huntington's disease: the nursing process. *Journal of Advanced Nursing, 6*:5, 377.

FINDLEY, L.J. & GRESTY, M.A. (1981) Tremor. *British Journal of Hospital Medicine, 26*:1, 16.

GUMPET, J. (1980) Tics, tremors and torsions. *The Practitioner, 224*:1345, 639.

LENMAN, J.A.R. (1982) Disorders of movement. *Hospital Update, 8*:1, 11.

PHILLIPS, D.H. (1982) *Living with Huntington's Disease*. London: Junction Books.

STIPE, J., WHITE, D. & VAN ARSDALE, E. (1979) Huntington's disease. *American Journal of Nursing, 79*:8, 1428.

THOMPSON, B. (1982) A case for sensitive care (Huntington's disease). *Nursing Mirror, 154*:18, 57.

19   Disorders of sensation

Sensations perceived may be physiological or pathological. Physiological sensations are appropriate to the stimulus, e.g. pain due to an insect sting or burn, but pathological sensations do not correspond to the stimulus. They may be diminished (hypalgesia), lost (anaesthesia), altered (dysaethesia) or accentuated, and sometimes occur without stimulus (paraesthesia). The lesions causing these abnormal sensations may be at any stage along the sensory pathways, i.e. the peripheral nerves, the nerve tracts in the spinal cord, the thalamus or the cerebral cortex.

NEURALGIAS

Neuralgia is an intense pain along the distribution of a nerve.

Trigeminal neuralgia

Trigeminal neuralgia (tic douloureux) is a distressing condition which generally occurs in elderly women and, although it may affect any of the divisions of the trigeminal nerve, it most commonly involves the maxillary branch. The paroxysms of sudden, severe pain, which last a few seconds, are produced by stimulating a 'trigger area' on the face. Eating, talking, shaving, brushing the teeth or a cold wind may each act as the stimulus, and the patient becomes frightened to continue these normal activities or to go outside. The attacks of pain often occur many times a day for several weeks and then disappear for months, but unfortunately their intensity and frequency generally increase. There is no obvious identifiable cause of trigeminal neuralgia, although it can occur in multiple sclerosis when an area of demyelination occurs within the brainstem.

Treatment

The most effective treatment available is carbamazepine (Tegretol) 200 mg twice daily, which can be increased to as much as 1600 mg daily. Unfortunately ataxia and drowsiness may occur as side-effects. If carbamazepine cannot be tolerated, phenytoin sodium (Epanutin) 100 mg three times a day is sometimes effective. Some patients fail to respond to drugs and in others the relief is not sustained. Some of these patients will benefit from a trial of trans-cutaneous nerve stimulation with the use of a mini-stimulator. Electrodes are placed on the patient's skin and a low-dose electrical current is produced by a portable, battery-operated, pulse generator. This can be performed on an out-patient basis.

If all else fails, surgical treatment may be indicated. This can take the form of the creation of a radio-frequency lesion by the generation of heat under detailed x-ray control and an intermittent general anaesthetic. Trigeminal thermocoagulation is a very safe procedure and is suitable for use on elderly female patients. The lesion can be carefully controlled to produce just the right amount of sensory deficit in the patient.

Treatment by injection of alcohol into the Gasserian (trigeminal) ganglion may be contemplated. This technique produces anaes-thesia in the distribution of the nerve, and stimulation of the trigger area no longer causes pain. The effect can last for up to 2 years and repetition of the injection may be sufficient to control the pain. Occasionally the anaesthesia is accompanied by an unpleasant burning sensation (anaesthesia dolorosa) which the patient finds as distressing as the original pain.

Division of the nerve root via a posterior fossa craniotomy was at one time the only surgical treatment available. However, with the advancement of safer and more effective techniques, this procedure is now rarely performed.

Related nursing skills. When patients are admitted to hospital with trigeminal neuralgia, they will probably be in very severe pain, which will not respond to conventional analgesia. It is imperative that any known trigger mechanism which will exacerbate the pain is avoided. A note should be made of these stimuli in the nursing history so that all personnel in the ward are aware of them. This information may need to be elicited from relatives in the event of the patient being unable to talk.

The patient should be nursed in a quiet, calm environment, and particular attention should be paid to nutrition. The patient may not have eaten for several days prior to admission, and the advice of the dietician should be sought. Many patients will manage some sort of diet with encouragement, although this is usually confined to clear soups and soft puddings.

The establishment of a proper drug regime, if this is the prescribed treatment, is essential in order to abolish the patient's pain. Tablets may need to be crushed in order that the patient may swallow them properly, and must be given at the correct times. Every opportunity should be taken to discuss the drug regime with the patient in order that he fully understands when the time comes for discharge. If the patient is to receive a course of transcutaneous nerve stimulation, an explanation of how the machine works must be given, and repeated on several occasions until he fully understands how to operate the machine safely. Prior to the application of the electrodes on or near the affected area, the patient washes the skin with some soap and warm water. The stimulator is then adjusted with the use of three controls until the pleasant buzzing feeling is obtained. Any reddening of the skin at the site of the electrodes can be avoided by alteration of their location at each session. Not every patient receives relief from the stimulator, and those who do not respond in the initial sessions require encouragement to pursue the treatment programme.

Patients who opt for surgical treatment, whether it is trigeminal thermocoagulation or a rhizotomy, will require routine pre- and postoperative nursing care with, in addition, special attention being paid to their eye care.

Some patients will experience a decrease of, or loss of, the corneal reflex and this will make the eye insensitive to any irritation which, if unheeded, will cause ulceration and keratitis. Diligent 2-hourly eye care needs to be performed and, before the patient goes home, he is instructed to continue with careful hygiene and twice-daily self-inspections of the eye, and urged that any redness must be reported to his doctor at once. The eye must be afforded extra protection by the addition of a clear plastic side-piece attached to the patient's own spectacles or to some plain glass ones.

Herpes zoster and post-herpetic neuralgia

The herpes zoster virus attacks the posterior root ganglion and presents as a vesicular rash along the distribution of the affected nerve, which is usually a trunk nerve from T6 to L1, or a division of the trigeminal nerve. Most patients are over 50 years of age and have no underlying disease; however, in young people it may be secondary to a chronic illness, e.g. carcinoma. The infection produces severe pain and, despite treatment with powerful analgesics and specific antiviral drugs, e.g. indoxuridine (Herpid), relief is often denied. The patient's natural response to immobilise the area must be discouraged because post-herpetic neuralgia may then result.

Post-herpetic neuralgia is particularly common in the elderly, and when the ophthalamic division of the trigeminal nerve has been involved, the burning, aching pain is unrelenting, and response to conventional analgesics or antidepressant therapy is poor. However, if amitriptyline (Tryptizol) 25 mg three times daily is combined with perphenazine (Fentazin) 2 mg three times daily, some relief may be achieved. Transcutaneous nerve stimulation may prove to be of help to some patients.

Glossopharyngeal neuralgia

Glossopharyngeal neuralgia is rare. The pain affects the throat, tongue and ear and is triggered off by swallowing. Treatment is to section the glossopharyngeal (IXth) cranial nerve via a posterior fossa approach.

Causalgia

Trauma often partially damages or completely divides a peripheral nerve, and such an injury may give rise to a severe burning pain associated with atrophy of the skin, hair loss and profuse sweating, i.e. causalgia. The skin is hypersensitive and the patient tries to protect it by not using the limb and by wrapping it in bandages.

Treatment of causalgia is often unsuccessful. Analgesics do not relieve the pain and although vigorous stimulation of the painful area, e.g. by rubbing with a rough towel or using a vibrator, is sometimes effective, starting treatment is so unpleasant that many patients refuse to continue. A sympathectomy may also afford some relief.

Phantom limb

Following amputation of a limb, the patient frequently feels that it is still present. This hallucination usually disappears in a few weeks, but if the limb has been amputated for a painful condition, e.g. ischaemic gangrene, the painful phantom may persist for many months, thereby suggesting that the pain pathways in the spinal cord and brain have become conditioned and no longer need external stimuli to produce the feeling of pain.

Thalamic lesions

Lesions of the thalamus initially cause contralateral loss of pain, but later produce a constant burning sensation. They usually result from an infarction, which often involves the internal capsule when a similar pain is experienced in the paralysed limbs. Phenytoin may afford some relief.

Syringomyelia

In this condition, which generally becomes apparent before the age of 30 years, the primary defect is in the drainage of the cerebro-spinal fluid from the fourth ventricle. A blockage in the foramen magnum area, usually due to herniation of the cerebellar tonsils, impedes the normal cerebrospinal fluid pathways and forces some of the fluid into the microscopic central canal, which extends from the medulla oblongata down the centre of the spinal cord (Fig. 19.1). The canal expands and usually ruptures into the substance of the cord (or, on rare occasions, into the medulla oblongata), form-ing a series of irregular cysts. Each cavity (syrinx), which usually occurs in the cervical region, becomes surrounded by fibrous tissue (gliosis; Fig. 19.2).

Because the central canal is in the central grey matter of the spinal cord, it is this region which suffers the earliest and greatest damage. The pain and temperature fibres of the arms, which cross through the cervical grey matter before ascending in the spinothalamic tract to the brain, are the first to be involved, and anaesthesia of the hands is therefore the initial symptom. The patient admits to not feeling pain from cuts or failing to realise that he has burnt his hand until he smells the scorching skin. As the syrinx expands, it com-presses the anterior horn cells, causing flaccid weakness and wasting of the muscles in the arms and hands, and the tendon reflexes are

(a)

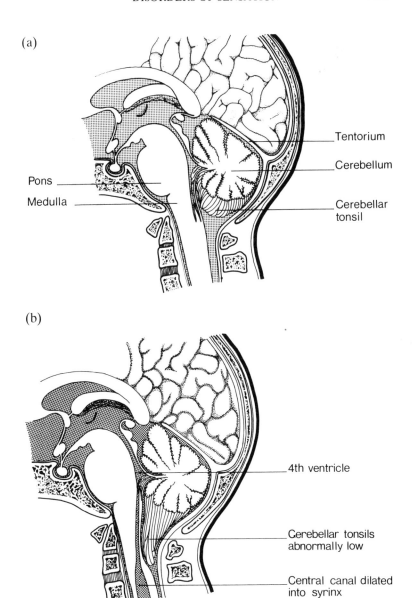

Tentorium

Cerebellum

Pons

Medulla

Cerebellar
tonsil

(b)

4th ventricle

Cerebellar tonsils
abnormally low

Central canal dilated
into syrinx

Fig. 19.1. *(a) Normal position of cerebellar tonsils compared with (b) cerebellar tonsils displaced in syringomyelia.*

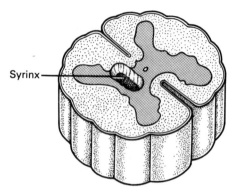

Fig. 19.2. *Syringomyelia.*

lost. Later, when the long tracts in the white matter are affected, the legs show spasticity.

When the medulla oblongata is involved, the condition is termed syringobulbia and its features are loss of pain and temperature sensation in the face, nystagmus and respiratory difficulties.

Investigations and treatment

Plain x-rays and myelography are used to assess the size and position of the cyst. Treatment is directed at improving the drainage of the cerebrospinal fluid from the fourth ventricle. The surgeon decompresses the abnormally situated cerebellar tonsils via a posterior fossa approach, and some improvement in sensation is often gained, although in some cases all that is achieved is an arrest of any deterioration.

Related nursing skills

The inability to feel pain or temperature in his hands requires the patient and those nursing him to watch his actions carefully so that injuries are reduced to a minimum. As further protection, the patient is advised to use insulated gloves when cooking and a cigarette holder when smoking. Splinting (light, very smooth wood supports are ideal) lessens trophic changes in the wasted and weakened hands, but eventually their strength is so reduced that the patient needs help in feeding, washing and dressing. Fortunately weakness in the legs is rarely severe, so mobility is retained.

In syringobulbia, a tracheostomy may be necessary if swallowing and coughing are severely disturbed, and death often results from a superimposed respiratory infection.

BROWN-SÉQUARD SYNDROME

Any lesion affecting one half of the spinal cord produces a characteristic picture of motor and sensory disturbances. Upper motor neurone weakness and loss of joint position and vibration sense occur below the lesion on the same side of the body, and loss of pain and temperature sensation is apparent on the opposite side of the body. This syndrome, named after the French physiologist C.E. Brown-Séquard, may result from an injury, an intramedullary or extramedullary tumour, or a plaque of multiple sclerosis.

TABES DORSALIS

Tabes dorsalis gives rise to a loss of sensation and also severe episodic pains.

PARAESTHESIAE

Paraesthesiae are usually 'pins and needles'. Sometimes they result from lesions in the posterior columns of the spinal cord or the peripheral nerves.

SPINAL CORD LESIONS

In young people, the commonest spinal lesion is multiple sclerosis (see Chapter 15); but in the elderly, subacute combined degeneration of the spinal cord, which can be cured if promptly diagnosed and treated, is more usual.

Subacute combined degeneration of the spinal cord

Severe vitamin B_{12} deficiency causes degeneration of the fibre tracts of the spinal cord. Involvement of the posterior columns produces loss of joint position sense and paraesthesiae. The latter, which is the commonest presenting symptom, starts in the feet and spreads (over a period of several weeks) to involve the legs and then the hands. Pyramidal tract signs subsequently develop, producing weakness, spasticity and extensor plantar responses. The deficiency of vitamin B_{12} also leads to a peripheral neuropathy (which contributes to the sensory disturbance), and sometimes dementia. Pernicious anaemia is frequently present, but similar syndromes are, on occasion, caused by folic acid deficiency.

Investigations include a blood count, bone marrow examination, estimation of serum B_{12}, and a Schilling test to determine if vitamin B_{12} is being absorbed.

Treatment

Following confirmation of the diagnosis, treatment with vitamin B_{12} injections is commenced, and must be continued for life. A common regime is hydroxocobalamin 1 mg by injection daily for 1 week, gradually reducing to a maintenance dose of 1 mg monthly. The neurological symptoms usually improve rapidly and in an early case complete recovery may be expected. In advanced deficiency, however, the results are poor, and if paraplegia has developed, mobility is rarely regained.

In such cases the nursing care for a paraplegic patient is necessary, as described in Chapter 17.

PERIPHERAL NERVE LESIONS

In the majority of cases, nerve degeneration (neuropathy) affects all the peripheral nerves (polyneuropathy), producing a symmetrical disturbance of function which is most marked in the feet. In some neuropathies, several individual nerves are attacked while others are spared (mononeuropathy multiplex), and sometimes only a single nerve is involved (mononeuropathy).

Causes of neuropathy

Metabolic causes. Diabetes mellitus produces a neuropathy in nearly all patients after 15 years, and is apparent as pins and needles and loss of sensation in the feet. On rare occasions, diabetic amyotrophy may occur. Other metabolically induced polyneuropathies can result from renal failure and porphyria, a disorder in which the neuropathy is precipitated when barbiturates are given.

Nutritional causes. Depletion in the vitamin B complex causes polyneuropathy which may be seen in beri-beri (vitamin B_1 deficiency), pernicious anaemia (vitamin B_{12} deficiency), malabsorption and poorly nourished alcoholics.

Toxins. Diphtheria, drugs (nitrofurantoin and vincristine) and heavy metals (lead, gold and mercury) act as toxins.

Malignant disease. Carcinoma of the bronchus sometimes produces a peripheral neuropathy, even when the carcinoma is too small to be detected.

Collagen disease. Systemic lupus erythematosus, polyarteritis nodosa and rheumatoid arthritis may produce a mononeuropathy multiplex.

Rare hereditary disorders. Peroneal muscular atrophy, where initially the muscles of the foot and then the lower leg become wasted, is an example. If the resultant footdrop is severe, the patient may benefit from special supports. The wasting process, which may also affect the muscles of the thighs and hands, is slowly progressive but life is not usually shortened. Diagnosis is made from nerve conduction studies and family history of similar disease.

Allergic responses. Serum sickness (reaction to an injection of serum or penicillin) may give rise to a brachial neuropathy.

Investigations

It is important to confirm the diagnosis and, if possible, to elicit its cause. Apart from examination of the cerebrospinal fluid and electromyogram studies, appropriate tests for the conditions previously listed are performed.

Traumatic lesions of peripheral nerves

Compression may damage the myelin sheaths of the nerve fibres, interrupting conduction of nerve impulses and therefore function of the nerve.

Upper limbs

Radial nerve palsy. The radial nerve may be compressed and stretched as a result of trauma caused by the prolonged use of crutches or as the drinker's arm hangs over the back of a chair during his drunken stupor — hence the term 'Saturday night palsy'. The resultant wrist drop requires no treatment, but a cock-up splint which keeps the wrist and fingers extended is sometimes helpful. The myelin sheath recovers rapidly and normal function is restored in a few weeks.

Carpal tunnel syndrome. Chronic compression of the median nerve in the carpal tunnel at the wrist produces episodes of paraesthesiae and pain in the thumb, index and middle fingers, and gradually causes atrophy of the thenar eminence. This condition is sometimes seen in people with intricate manual jobs, e.g. dressmaking or watch repairing. Treatment by splinting and local hydrocortisone injection may help, but usually decompression by a complete division of the carpal ligament is required. The indication for surgery is either when the pain begins to wake the patient from sleep or when there is wasting of the thenar eminence. Following surgery, the patient's hand is well bandaged and supported on a pillow or in a sling (which can be made out of a roller towel pinned to hold the forearm in a vertical position) attached to an intravenous infusion stand. He is encouraged to move his fingers frequently, and on the first postoperative day the wound is redressed in a light bandage which the patient must keep dry when he goes home, returning on the tenth day after surgery for removal of his sutures. The results are good.

Ulnar nerve. The ulnar nerve may be compressed at the elbow, causing wasting of the small muscles of the hand and sensory disturbance in the little finger and border of the hand.

Lower limbs

Wallerian degeneration. More severe trauma, including division of the nerve in a lacerating injury, results in Wallerian degeneration. The nerve axons distal to the injury degenerate, as do their myelin sheaths. If the nerve remains continuous, or a divided nerve is sutured, regeneration of the nerve fibres starts a few days after the injury and growth is at the rate of 1 mm/day. Recovery, especially after division of the nerve, is often incomplete and takes many months. There is total anaesthesia in the distribution of the nerve and the patient must be warned to take special care to avoid burning or otherwise injuring himself, e.g. when smoking. This is especially important in lesions of the median nerve because the thumb and index finger are at risk. Sometimes tendon transposition operations are needed to improve the function of limbs when injured nerves fail to regenerate.

Femoral nerve. The femoral nerve may be damaged during surgery of the pelvis. Treatment consists of bed rest; most cases respond spontaneously, although decompressive surgery may be contemplated.

Sciatic nerve. Following a difficult labour, some women develop sensory loss of the innervated area and footdrop, and complain of pain across the small of the back due to compression of the sciatic nerve. Other causes may include injection of medication into the nerve, or pelvic fractures.

Common peroneal nerve. The common peroneal nerve may be compressed during surgery, the patient developing footdrop and sensory loss of the innervated area. Treatment is conservative.

Posterior tibial nerve (tarsal tunnel syndrome). This is the equivalent to the carpal tunnel syndrome, but occurs in the ankle, producing pain in the toes and soles of the feet. Treatment is similar to that for carpal tunnel syndrome.

Plantar nerve. Repeated trauma to the medial aspect of the sole, as may occur in 'joggers', may produce a burning pain in the heel and loss of sensory function.

CORTICAL SENSORY DISTURBANCES

Lesions of the parietal lobe may produce a sensory deficit which prevents fine discrimination. Although pain and touch are still felt on the side opposite to the lesion, the patient is unable to identify objects placed on his hand or numbers drawn on the skin. The patient may also ignore the affected half of his body, and this defect, which makes him accident prone, is called sensory inattention. It can be tested by giving a stimulus to each hand, one of which the patient will disregard. When sensory inattention occurs in association with a hemiplegia due to a stroke, rehabilitation is very difficult and injuries may be sustained because the limbs are neglected and the patient is insufficiently aware of his weakness and sensory loss.

Related nursing skills

The sensory system forms an important part of the body's defence, and any compromise leaves the patient with an increased chance of being injured. The nurse must be aware of this vulnerability and construct an effective teaching plan for the patient.

The patient must avoid coming into contact with extremes of temperature, which may inflict a lot of damage before he realises that he is in danger. Skin care is important and regular inspections of the denervated area should be performed to ensure that no breakdown has occurred, e.g. as may be caused by badly fitting shoes.

The patient with footdrop may require a toe spring and/or a caliper to mobilise, and if the neuropathy affects the arm, immobilisation of the affected limb with the use of light-weight splints or plaster of Paris casts may be indicated. The colour and warmth of the immobilised limb should be checked, and the patient instructed that if he experiences any discomfort or swelling, he should notify his doctor. The process of recovering function of a limb can be slow and frustrating for the patient and his family, and they should be given an opportunity to vent their feelings.

A marked sensory disturbance in the hands makes it difficult for the patient to hold small objects, but by padding the handles of implements, e.g. eating utensils, increased independence can be achieved.

FURTHER READING

GUIN, P.R. (1982) Radiofrequency lesions — a treatment for trigeminal neuralgia. *Journal of Neurosurgical Nursing, 14*:3, 192.

SMITH, C. (1980) Peripheral nerve lesions — 1. *Nursing Times, 76*:47, 2057.

SMITH, C. (1980) Peripheral nerve lesions —2. The upper limbs. *Nursing Times, 76*:48, 2116.

SMITH, C. (1980) Peripheral nerve lesions —3. The lower limbs. *Nursing Times, 76*:49, 2159.

20   Dementia

Dementia is deterioration (frequently permanent) in intellectual function which is sometimes classified according to age (presenile before and senile after 65 years). It is usually chronic and progressive, although with little change from day to day. The conscious level is not altered.

In comparison, temporary fluctuating disturbances of mental function, often with clouding of conscious level (confusion); occur in many acute illnesses (e.g. infectious diseases of the nervous system or elsewhere when the temperature is very high), situations where the oxygen supply to the brain is reduced (e.g. heart failure and intoxications, in particular by alcohol or sleeping pills). In all these conditions the mental state (which is most commonly upset in the very young and elderly) returns to normal when the underlying disorder has resolved.

Although most cases of dementia have an irreversible cause, all patients are investigated in order to exclude any treatable condition.

CAUSES OF DEMENTIA

Causes of dementia may be classified according to whether they are irreversible or treatable.

Irreversible causes

Primary cerebral atrophy

Primary cerebral atrophy is the commonest cause. This may be in the form of Alzheimer's disease, where generalised atrophy of the cerebral cortex occurs, or Pick's disease, where only the fronto-temporal lobes are affected. In both cases the age of onset is usually between 40 and 60 years, and apart from generalised intellectual impairment, focal neurological signs, e.g. hemiparesis and dysphasia, may develop. The patient has little or no insight into his deterioration and may continue at work, making frequent mistakes.

Later on he may tend to wander from the house and be unable to find his way back.

Huntington's chorea

See p. 245.

Jakob–Creutzfeldt disease

Jakob–Creutzfeldt disease is a very rare condition which causes rapid progressive dementia associated with rigidity and jerky involuntary movements. It is thought to be due to a 'slow virus' that becomes apparent in middle or old age.

Cerebral vascular disease

Repeated strokes may cause dementia and these patients also demonstrate neurological deficits.

Head injury

A severe accident may damage so many neurones that permanent loss of intellectual function results. Repeated minor trauma eventually has the same outcome and is the cause of the 'punch drunk' boxer.

Treatable causes

Cerebral tumours

Any slow-growing tumour in a 'silent area' of the brain may present with dementia and no focal signs. Mood changes, especially euphoria, suggest a lesion in the frontal lobes.

Hydrocephalus

Obstruction to the drainage of cerebrospinal fluid from the ventricles usually causes raised intracranial pressure, with headache and vomiting. Sometimes, when the blockage occurs slowly, the brain compensates for the increase in the ventricle size by tissue shrinkage, which mainly takes place in the cortex. Dementia becomes apparent, but signs of raised intracranial pressure do not develop. This phenomenon is generally seen when adhesions (usually caused by bacterial meningitis or blood from a spontaneous or traumatic subarachnoid haemorrhage, but occasionally of unknown origin) obstruct the cerebrospinal fluid flow in the subarachnoid space.

Deficiency disorders

Vitamin B_{12}, nicotinic acid and thiamine deficiencies can all present as dementia. The last two will present as an acute delirium; the thiamine-deficient delirium is termed Wernicke's encephalopathy. The patient demonstrates marked disturbances and will confabulate to cover up for this. Vitamin B_{12} deficiency may or may not occur with an associated anaemia. Serum vitamin B_{12} is very low.

Metabolic disorders

Hypothyroidism produces slowing of mental functions, and dementia may be the most marked feature. Chronic liver disease and hypoglycaemia may manifest themselves with dementia.

Syphilis

General paralysis of the insane is rarely seen now, but in the early stages can be cured with penicillin.

INVESTIGATION OF PATIENTS WITH DEMENTIA

A range of investigations is available in order to determine which type of dementia the patient may have.

Preliminary investigations will consist of obtaining a full history of the patient's illness and performing a neurological examination. Psychometric assessment can indicate the severity of the dementia, and the patient's score in different tests may reveal which parts of the hemispheres are most markedly affected. Electroencephalography may demonstrate an unsuspected focal lesion, e.g. a tumour or subdural haematoma, or generalised reduction in electrical activity consistent with primary cerebral atrophy.

A CT scan will demonstrate a tumour or any hydrocephalus,

while a radio-isotope scan will demonstrate an increased uptake in the presence of a tumour. Further selective investigations may be required to establish a particular dementia. These include serum electrolytes, measurement of vitamin B_{12} levels, Wassermann reactions, a full haematological picture, thyroid function and examination of the cerebrospinal fluid.

MEDICAL TREATMENT

Treatment of dementia depends on the underlying cause; unfortunately irreversible types are not treatable. Where there is a tumour, this may be amenable to surgical intervention; hydrocephalus is treated with a shunting procedure. Deficiency disorders require replacement of the depleted substance. Syphilis is treated with penicillin.

Related nursing skills

These patients act irrationally at times, are often forgetful, and may display emotional lability by fluctuating between weeping and laughing in response to comments in conversation. The nurse, in her efforts to try to keep the patient content and behaving in a tolerable manner, must show decorum and answer the patient's questions sensibly. Demented patients have a tendency to wander off and become lost once they have left the ward. In the most severe cases, the patient cannot find his way to the bathroom or back to his own bed. The nurse must keep a careful watch on the patient's movements and, when necessary, gently guide him back to his bed or chair. It is useful to keep the patient's bed in the same position and to keep his environment unaltered in order to aid his orientation.

Although loss of sphincter control is not usually an early feature (it may occur in some tumours and in communicating hydrocephalus), the patient becomes incontinent and unable to dress or feed himself in the late stages of a dementing illness. In these circumstances full nursing care will be required.

It should be borne in mind that the patient's confusion is often exacerbated during the night, and extra precautions may be required in terms of closer observation, special equipment and staffing levels.

It is important to remember that the relatives of a demented patient will be distressed to see both the mental and physical deterioration, and they should be reassured that the patient is not aware of his loss of mental faculties. Care by the nurse not to treat him as a fool or child will reduce anxieties and help the family to retain their motivation in looking after him. Relatives often find it hard to accept that most forms of dementia are progressive, and require frequent confirmation that no therapeutic possibility has been ignored. With adequate help from the social services, the patient's family can often keep him in the protected environment of his home for several years, but eventually institutional care in a psychiatric or psychogeriatric unit is usually needed.

FURTHER READING

COWIE, V. (1980) Old before your time (presenile dementia). *Nursing Mirror, 152*:7, 44.

CYBYK, M.E. (1980) Alzheimer's disease. *Nursing Times, 76*:7, 280.

GRAY, A. (1982) Old before their time (Alzheimer's disease). *Nursing Mirror, 154*:2, 39.

IVESON-IVESON, J. (1981) Senile dementia. *Nursing Mirror, 153*:12, 34.

KENNEDY, E. (1981) Rosie . . . our Rosie (senile dementia). *Nursing Mirror, 153*:20, 49.

21 Spina bifida and hydrocephalus

SPINA BIFIDA

At a very early stage in development, the nervous system consists of a layer of tissue on the dorsal surface of the embryo. This strip rolls into a tube (the neural tube), the anterior end of which enlarges, folds and forms outgrowths, and eventually develops into the brain. A bony casing (the skull and vertebral column) then forms round the system. Malformations in this complex process of development may occur, and the most severe cause the fetus to die in the uterus.

The commonest abnormalities arise while the vertebral canal is developing and as the tube formation of the spinal cord is completed. The most frequent sites are the lumbar and occipital regions. Spina bifida is the failure of the vertebral arch to fuse in the midline. This defect may be small and concealed, or extensive and visible (Fig. 21.1).

Spina bifida occulta

Occulta means hidden, and often there are no outward indications of the bony defect in spina bifida occulta, which may only come to light following x-rays and palpation of the spine. However, it may be suspected because of slight external abnormalities, e.g. overlying dimpled deposits of fat or tufts of hair. A track may pass from the dimple to the spinal canal, allowing the entry of infection, or it may lead to a lipoma or dermoid cyst which acts as a spinal tumour. Sometimes there is a malformation of the lowest part of the spinal cord (the conus medullaris), which causes bladder disturbances in adult life. The tethered cord which becomes stretched because it does not grow as much as the vertebral column may be surgically released.

Spina bifida cystica

The defect in the vertebral arch is wide and often involves several

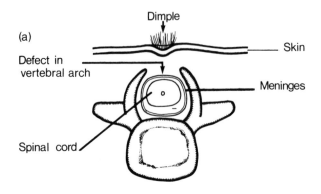

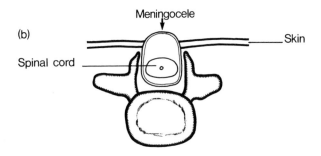

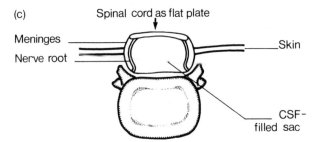

Fig. 21.1. *Varieties of spina bifida: (a) spina bifida occulta, (b) meningocele, and (c) myelomeningocele.*

vertebrae in spina bifida cystica. There is also an imperfection of the skin, so that the meninges or even the spinal cord and nerve roots tie on the surface, conditions known as meningocele and myelomeningocele respectively. All patients with a meningocele and some of those with a myelomeningocele are referred for surgical closure of the abnormality within 24 hours of birth.

Related nursing skills

Preoperative care

The defect is covered with a sterile moist dressing and the baby is nursed prone in an incubator. His spine is x-rayed and the paediatrician examines the site and size of the lesion and assesses the neurological damage. The physiotherapist may be requested to perform a muscle assessment survey. If the spinal cord is involved, paralysis of the legs and of anal and urethral sphincters is common. Other congenital abnormalities, in particular talipes equinovarus (clubfoot), dislocation of the hips and hydrocephalus, are frequently associated with spina bifida. The prompt detection of hydrocephalus, which may not develop until after the spinal lesion is closed, is ensured by daily measurements of the head circumference in all spina bifida babies.

The surgeon will discuss the problems with the baby's parents, outlining the degree of disability and the possible outcome of surgery. Any future problems or complications which it is reasonably thought that the baby may suffer from will also be sympathetically explained. The fact that their baby has a major abnormality is very distressing for parents, and they will find it hard to accept. Sympathetic support from medical and nursing staff is very important.

If consent is obtained for operation, the baby will be prepared in the usual manner and taken to theatre. The operation involves dissecting the meninges and nervous structures from the skin and closing the defect by mobilising skin flaps.

Postoperative care

The baby is received into a prewarmed incubator and nursed prone without a napkin. Some centres advocate the use of a sling to keep pressure off the wound site. Dribbling incontinence of urine and faeces may occur, and keeping the skin dry, clean and free from excoriation requires diligent nursing care. The dressing is changed if it becomes soiled, and in view of the high risk of wound infections and meningitis, antibiotics may be given prophylactically. Gentle expression of the bladder will help to prevent stagnation of urine and urinary tract infections. The sutures are removed 10 days postoperatively and, provided the wound has healed, the baby is discharged.

If the spinal cord and nerve roots are involved in the defect, the operation to close the spina bifida is only the first of a large number of surgical procedures that the child will require to control hydrocephalus, correct orthopaedic deformities and manage urinary incontinence. Mental retardation is common, and many patients die in early infancy or childhood; only a few have slight disabilities, and clearly the burden on the majority of parents who bring up a child with spina bifida is considerable. The nurse can help the parents in their task. During the postoperative period the parents can aid in the child's nursing care, which allows the nurse to participate in parent teaching. Points which will be covered include feeding difficulties, how to hold the baby properly, and comfortably, express the baby's bladder, perform passive range of movement exercises and take care of the skin, emphasising the need to prevent pressure sores and of the dangers of decreased sensation.

Parents will receive community support from their general practitioner, health visitor and community nurse, and some may benefit from membership of the Association for Spina Bifida and Hydrocephalus which provides a welfare and advisory service.

HYDROCEPHALUS

The cerebrospinal fluid

The cerebral ventricles (Fig. 21.2) and the subarachnoid space surrounding the brain and spinal cord are filled with cerebrospinal fluid. The cerebrospinal fluid assists in regulating intracranial pressure and cerebral metabolism and, most importantly, acts as a cushion preventing injury of the brain against the skull during movement of the head. It is produced by a tuft of capillaries covered with ependyma (choroid plexus) in each of the ventricles, through

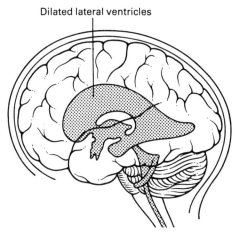

Dilated lateral ventricles

Fig. 21.2. *Hydrocephalus.*

the foramen of Munro to the third ventricle and then down the aqueduct of Sylvius to the fourth ventricle, and enters the cisterna magna. Some cerebrospinal fluid then circulates round the spinal cord, but eventually it all flows upwards. The subarachnoid space is narrow at the level of the tentorium, but normally the fluid flows through this region and then over the surface of the cerebral hemisphere to the arachnoid villi. The cerebrospinal fluid is returned to the vascular system by being transported through the cells of the villi into the venous sinuses.

The total volume of cerebrospinal fluid is about 150 ml and of this, 30–50 ml is in the ventricular system. Obstruction of any of the narrow channels through which the cerebrospinal fluid has to pass will create a dam in its flow and lead to dilatation of the ventricles above the blockage; this is termed hydrocephalus.

A tumour may block the aqueduct, the third or fourth ventricle, adhesions may obstruct the exits from the fourth ventricle or the entrance to the subarachnoid space at the tentorium. The resultant symptoms depend on the speed at which the obstruction develops, whether compensation occurs with other routes of cerebrospinal fluid absorption, and the age of the patient.

Hydrocephalus in infants

In infants the sutures (joints between the bones of the skull) have not fused. When the flow of cerebrospinal fluid is obstructed, the intraventricular pressure rises and the ventricles dilate. The raised pressure causes the fontanelles to bulge and the sutures to widen. The vault of the skull enlarges, making the face appear small in comparison. Drowsiness, irritability, a high-pitch cry and vomiting are further features.

The reason for hydrocephalus in infancy may be congenital abnormalities, e.g. stenosis of the aqueduct, or an abnormally low position of the cerebellar tonsils which obstruct the exit from the fourth ventricle (Arnold–Chiari malformation).

Post-meningitic adhesions around the exit of the fourth ventricle are also an important cause. If an infant has a condition which increases the risk of developing hydrocephalus, e.g. spina bifida, regular measurements of the head circumference and comparison with a graph of normal values will lead to early detection and prompt treatment of the hydrocephalus (Fig. 21.3).

If the hydrocephalus is not relieved at an early stage, permanent damage ensues. The papilloedema caused by the raised intracranial pressure may progress to blindness, and the compression of the cerebral tissue by the expanded ventricles may lead to mental retardation and spastic weakness of the limbs. The majority of these patients succumb to infection, to which they are particularly prone, while still in childhood.

Hydrocephalus in older children and adults

Once the sutures have fused, the skull becomes a rigid box and the distended ventricular system behaves as a space-occupying lesion. Headaches, vomiting, papilloedema and drowsiness develop. Sometimes obstruction of the cerebrospinal fluid flow is incomplete, or an alternative route of absorption develops, i.e. the hydrocephalus is compensated. In these cases the intracranial pressure is often normal, and progressive dementia is the presenting symptom.

Investigations

X-ray of the skull in infants shows widening of the sutures and thinning of the bones. In adults, the dorsum sellae behind the pituitary fossa is frequently eroded by raised intracranial pressure.

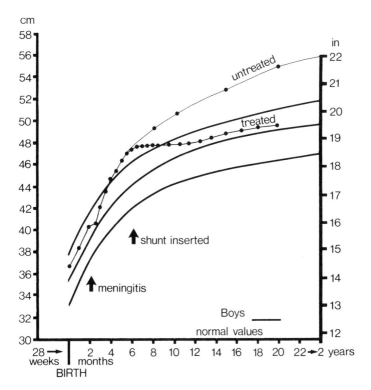

HEAD CIRCUMFERENCE

Fig. 21.3. *Head circumference chart.*

If the blockage is within the ventricular system, it stops the cerebrospinal fluid from communicating with the subarachnoid space, i.e. non-communicating hydrocephalus; but if the obstruction is beyond this juncture, i.e. the tentorial opening, the hydrocephalus is termed communicating.

The presence of dilated ventricles will be confirmed by CT scanning, and ventricular isotope scanning, involving the injection of indium and DPTA via a lumbar or cisternal puncture, will outline the pathways.

Treatment

If the cerebellar tonsils are blocking the exit from the fourth ventricle, decompression of the foramen magnum may cure the condition. Also, on rare occasions, it is possible to excise an obstructing tumour, although it is usually necessary to alleviate the hydrocephalus before embarking on major intracranial surgery. Temporary relief is obtained by ventricular drainage, but frequently a more permanent method of bypassing the obstruction is needed. The flow of cerebrospinal fluid is either diverted within its own system (internal shunt) or drained into another body cavity (external shunt).

Internal shunt

Torkildsen's operation may be performed for non-communicating hydrocephalus. A Silastic (silicone-rubber) tube is inserted into the occipital horn of one of the lateral ventricles via a burr hole, and the other end is placed into the cisterna magna, so bypassing the obstruction (Fig. 21.4). A duplicate procedure will be needed if the cerebrospinal outflow from both ventricles is impeded.

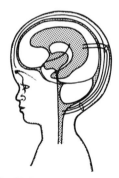

Fig. 21.4. *Torkildsen's operation.*

External shunt

The ventriculo-atrial shunt (Fig. 21.5) is for both types of hydro-cephalus, and is now used in the treatment of the majority of patients. A Silastic catheter is inserted, with the proximal end in a lateral ventricle (usually right) and the distal end in the right atrium. At some point in the catheter a one-way valve is placed to allow cerebrospinal fluid to pass from the cerebral ventricle to the heart, but to prevent blood flowing in the opposite direction. A valve

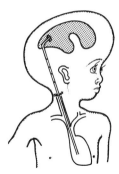

Fig. 21.5. *Ventriculo-atrial shunt and position of a Spitz–Holter valve in a hydrocephalic child.*

made to open at high pressure (100–200 mmH₂O) may be inserted to relieve intraventricular obstruction, and one that will release at a low pressure (40–60 mmH₂O) may be used in cases of communicating hydrocephalus. Alternatively, the surgeon may choose a valve that releases at medium pressure (60–100 mmH₂O) for either type of hydrocephalus. An antisyphon valve, which closes when the intracranial pressure falls below zero (i.e. when the patient stands), prevents excessive drainage of cerebrospinal fluid and may be used in series with a low-, medium- or high-pressure valve.

The ventricular catheter has a number of side holes, and is introduced into the frontal horn of the right lateral ventricle through a parietal burr hole and secured by a suture. The valve is positioned so that it lies behind the ear. The venous catheter is then attached and passed under the skin to a further incision in the side of the neck. Next the surgeon dissects out a vessel that drains into the external jugular vein, inserts the catheter and threads it via the external jugular vein and the superior vena cava into the right atrium. The venous catheter, which has a single end-hole to prevent blood clotting in it, is then anchored by ligatures round the vein in the neck.

The ventriculo-peritoneal shunt is used for both types of hydrocephalus. The distal section of the catheter is passed through a subcutaneous track in the chest wall and the end, which has several side holes, lies in the peritoneal cavity.

Ideally, a shunt continues to work indefinitely, but failure due to blockage at the ventricular end or blood clotting in the atrial tip (or adhesions forming round a peritoneal catheter) is common and necessitates revision. As the hydrocephalic child grows, the atrial catheter becomes too short to reach the heart, and regular revisions, the first of which is usually needed between the ages of 18 months and 3 years, are undertaken.

Related nursing skills

Preoperative care

After the patient has been investigated, the most suitable type of shunt is chosen. The procedure is explained and the consent obtained (from the patient if responsible, but otherwise from the next of kin). The appropriate areas are shaved (bearing in mind that the shunt has two ends), and the patient is prepared in the routine preoperative manner.

The intracranial pressure is often very high, and if so the patient may be drowsy, vomiting and dehydrated. Accurate neurological observations are essential to detect any deterioration in the patient's condition which may change an elective procedure into an emergency. Careful recording of fluid balance is also important; the patient may be given intravenous fluid to counteract the effects of vomiting.

Postoperative care

The shunt should work immediately, and some improvement in the patient's conscious level will be seen quickly. The nurse must continually watch for evidence of shunt failure. Drowsiness is a constant feature and is accompanied by further signs of raised intracranial pressure, usually headache and vomiting in the adult and a tense, bulging fontanelle in the child. Measurement of the head circumference is continued postoperatively. If a valved shunt has been used, it might be considered worthwhile to attempt to pump it to overcome the obstruction; however, this is only performed under medical direction.

Failure to fill the valve indicates a persistent block at the proximal end, and an inability to empty it suggests a fault at the distal end.

Other postoperative complications may include pressure necrosis at the back of the child's head; this is due to the inability of the child to move his head freely due to its enlarged size, and therefore frequent changes of head position are necessary. When lifting the child, always lift and support the head first. A shunt is a foreign body and any infection of it may be impossible to eradicate. Great care must be taken with all procedures, especially dressing the wounds, to avoid introducing infection. The head sutures and those that anchor the catheter are removed at the time specified by the surgeon.

Prognosis

Children

The susceptibility of these children to infection (in particular meningitis) means that most do not survive into adult life, and those that do usually have significant mental and/or physical disability.

The parents of a hydrocephalic child require a great deal of help and support from both hospital and community staff in facing the situation of caring for, and possibly losing, a handicapped child.

Membership of the Association for Spina Bifida and Hydrocephalus may be of benefit to the parents; it provides numerous services to assist the carers.

Adults

Even though the cause of hydrocephalus cannot always be cured, e.g. a tumour obstructing the aqueduct, shunting may relieve most of the patient's symptoms and allow several more months or years of normal activities. When communicating hydrocephalus has led to dementia, the results of treatment are very variable.

FURTHER READING

ANDERSON, E.M. & SPAIN, B. (1977) *The Child with Spina Bifida*. London: Methuen.

BALDRIDGE, J. (1982) Arnold–Chiari malformation. *Journal of Neurosurgical Nursing, 14*:4, 162.

BRUNNER, L.S. & SUDDARTH, D.S. (1981) *Lippincott Manual of Paediatric Nursing*, 2nd edn. London: Harper and Row.

GARROW, D. (1981) A loving thing to do. *Nursing Mirror, 152*:18, 27.

HOSKING, G. (1982) Treating the untreatable (spina bifida). *Nursing Mirror, 154*:24, 31.

SACHARIN, R.M. (1980) *Principles of Paediatric Nursing*, 1st edn., p. 190. Edinburgh: Churchill Livingstone.

STARK, G.D. (1977) *Spina Bifida, Problems and Management*. Oxford: Blackwell Scientific.
THORNS, S. (1982) Controversy, treatment and care. *Nursing Mirror, 154*:24, 32.
THORNS, S. (1982) The best possible start. *Nursing Mirror, 154*:24, 33.
ZACHRAY, R. (1981) 'To let live' or 'cause to die'. *Nursing Mirror, 152*:18, 27.

USEFUL ADDRESS

The Association for Spina Bifida and Hydrocephalus
Tavistock House North
Tavistock Square
London WC1

22   Pain relief

Appreciation of pain is one of the body's defences against harmful stimuli. Lack of pain perception can lead to repeated minor injury with eventual mutilation, e.g. loss of fingers in syringomyelia, or corneal ulceration following damage to the trigeminal nerve. Some diseases cause continuous severe pain (e.g. carcinoma invading bone), and others alter sensation so that any slight, non-harmful stimulus provokes pain (e.g. causalgia and trigeminal neuralgia). This excessive perception of pain prevents rest and demoralises even the most stoical people so that they can think of little else except obtaining relief from their persistent discomfort.

Before examining methods of relieving pain, we must look further at the mechanism and perceptions of pain. This is only a very brief outline and the reader is recommended to consult with a specialised pain textbook for further information. Over the years, several researchers have postulated as to the true mechanism of pain, and many ideas have been produced. One theory which has received a favourable response is the gate control theory, in which it is stated that stimulation of the large non-pain-bearing myelinated nerve fibres somehow suppresses pain impulses along the small unmyelinated fibres by closing a synaptic 'gate'. Whether the brain perceives pain or not depends on the number of impulses bombarding the 'gate' at any one time, which in turn determines whether the 'gate' is open or closed. This is a simplified version of the theory, which does not meet with universal agreement.

Perception of pain is a complex issue, having both physical and psychological aspects, which will vary from person to person. Different social and cultural backgrounds will produce differing attitudes towards pain, as do also sex and age. Many people's perception of pain will rely on a past experience of a painful event in their life. Many nurses still have difficulty in coming to terms with the patient who complains of pain, which is resolved merely by giving the patient analgesic drugs or even withholding them if they do not think that the patient has a pain. The concept that a patient is bound to have more pain following major surgery than he would have following a minor procedure no longer holds true. The patients with whom we are concerned are those suffering unremitting pain from various causes, either known or unknown. If the cause is known, it will be of benefit to the patient to remove it, e.g. in an inflammatory disorder drugs would be given to reduce the inflammation as well as measures to reduce the pain.

DRUG THERAPY

Analgesics vary in potency and are chosen according to the doctor's assessment of the severity of the patient's pain. The narcotic analgesics, which are generally the most powerful, all lead to addiction and therefore their use is confined to those situations where severe pain is likely to be of short duration, e.g. following injury or operation, or where the patient's life expectancy is limited. In terminal cases, the regular administration of a small quantity of analgesia before the action of the previous dose has abated is more effective in controlling distressing symptoms than irregular large amounts given when the patient complains of pain. Other drugs, such as hypnotics antidepressants and tranquillisers, may be used in conjunction with analgesics.

COUNTER STIMULATION

Counter stimulation of the painful region with heat, cold or vibration may produce relief, although this will only be temporary.

If these methods fail to alleviate the pain or the patient is in severe discomfort from a condition which does not threaten life, it may be feasible to interrupt the pain impulses between the diseased part and the area of the brain where pain is perceived.

ELECTRICAL STIMULATION

Transcutaneous nerve stimulation. This is performed by applying two external electrodes over the painful area which are connected up to a portable, battery-operated pulse generator producing a pleasant low-dose electrical current. The stimulator has a moderate success rate, and little or no harmful side-effects. It can only be used under professional supervision, although once the patient is proficient in the use of the machine, he may be given one to use at home.

Peripheral nerve stimulation. This is a similar method to that used for transcutaneous nerve stimulation, except that the electrodes are implanted.

Dorsal column stimulation. An electrode is implanted within the extradural space above the segment of pain. Wires are led out to a radio-frequency receiver over which the patient has control. A continuous or intermittent stimulus can be provided to obtain optimum relief.

Cerebral stimulation. This is an advanced procedure in which stereotactic techniques are employed to stimulate the paraventricular grey matter situated between the third ventricle and the thalamus. Stimulation of this area is thought to release encephalins, which, it is suggested, constitute the body's own endogenous pain-relieving mechanism.

SURGICAL PROCEDURES

Peripheral nerve section. A peripheral nerve may, if its motor function is not important, be interrupted by an injection of local anaesthetic, or destroyed by phenol, e.g. an intercostal nerve can be injected via the intercostal space in the paraspinal region for relief of pain caused by bronchial carcinoma invading the chest wall.

Rhizotomy. If it is important to preserve motor function, the sensory roots are divided within the vertebral canal. Segments above and below the pain segment also need to be divided for effective relief. However, this type of procedure will deprive the affected areas of all forms of sensation, thus exposing the patient to the danger of injury.

Cordotomy. When pain fibres enter the spinal cord, they cross to the opposite side and ascend in the lateral spinothalamic tract. This is near the surface of the cord and can be divided (spinothalamic cordotomy) without injury to other fibre tracts. There is loss of pain and temperature sensation below the level of the lesion (T2 for leg pain, C1–2 for arm pain) on the opposite side of the body, but light touch and proprioception are preserved so the limbs remain protected and useful.

The results of this operation are good if the pain is unilateral, e.g. phantom pain following an amputation. Midline or bilateral pain requires bilateral cordotomies, and these frequently produce sphincter disturbance (the fibres to the bladder lie just under the spinothalamic tract) and spasticity of the legs.

Tractotomy.   The pain fibres may be divided at a higher level, i.e. in the medulla or midbrain.

Thalamotomy.   All the pain fibres have a synapse in the thalamus, and stereotaxic destructive lesions in the appropriate area may be helpful.

Pituitary neuroadenolysis.   This involves the injecting of alcohol via the transphenoidal route into the pituitary fossa, destroying the pituitary gland. Its use is indicated in reducing pain from hormone-dependent tumours of the body.

RELATED NURSING SKILLS

General measures

The role of the nurse is very important in the care of patients with chronic pain. A friendly and sympathetic attitude — pausing for a chat, making sure that the patient is lying comfortably and offering analgesics — will frequently help the patient to bear his pain with less distress.

The response to the same painful stimulus varies in different patients from 'just a slight twinge' to 'severe anguish'. The nurse, who spends more time with the patient than the doctor, can help to assess the individual's susceptibility to pain and the type of analgesic he will require. Confused or dysphasic patients may be unable to express their discomfort, and occasionally a patient suffers in silence because he does not want to bother anyone; but careful observation of each patient's expression and behaviour usually indicates if he is in discomfort. Pain tends to have a depressing effect, the patient usually wanting to lie quietly alone.

Pain in the night seems worse than pain during the day. There are no distractions, sleep is elusive and the hours of darkness seem unending. This is often an ideal time to comfort and talk to the patient. Some patients who cannot bear the thought of perpetual pain confess to suicidal thoughts, and these should be reported to the sister or the medical staff. A priest or chaplain can often comfort such patients and the medical social worker may be able to solve any domestic worries.

Specific measures

It is important when administering drugs that they are given on time and in the correct dose. The regulations pertaining to the safe keeping of controlled drugs must be adhered to. The nurse should establish that the patient is able to take his medication, and patients who find tablets difficult to take or a suspension distasteful will have to be provided with a suitable alternative. Many analgesics can have unpleasant side-effects, and these need to be countered with nursing intervention and further medication. If cold or hot applications are being used to act as a counter stimulant, care will be needed when applying these extremes of temperature, particularly in the patient with impaired sensation.

Careful instruction in the use of the electrical machinery involved in transcutaneous, peripheral and dorsal column stimulation will be required. All patients will learn the techniques at various rates and should not be left alone until they are confident and competent at operating the stimulator. The tingling produced should be a pleasant sensation, and over-stimulation will lead to irritation of the skin under the electrodes. This can be avoided by rotating the position of the electrodes at each session. A family member should also be instructed in the use of the machine, and it is emphasised that the stimulator is for the patient's sole use.

Following cordotomy, the patient is closely observed for respiratory depression. An apnoea monitor should be kept *in situ* for 24–48 hours. Some centres advocate that the patient receives continuous oxygen over the same period via nasal cannulae as a precaution. Avoidance of any respiratory depressant drugs is necessary, and the patient is observed for signs of hypoxia, i.e. he may become disorientated or display bizarre behaviour.

FURTHER READING

ALLAN, D. (1981) The use of transcutaneous nerve stimulation in patients with severe pain. *Nursing Times, 77*:40, 1721.

CHAPMAN, C. (1979) Treating the patient as an individual. *Nursing (UK)*, 1st series, *1*, 3

CONDON, P. (1980) Pain relief — the nurse's role. *Nursing Times, 76*:24, 1052.

CROW, R. (1979) The nature of pain. *Nursing (UK)*, 1st series, *1*, 6.

HANNINGTON-KIFF, F.G. (1979) The mechanism of pain. *Nursing (UK)*, 1st series, *1*, 12.

HAYWARD, J. (1979) Psychological and social aspects. *Nursing (UK),* 1st series, *1*, 21.

HUNT, J.M. (1979) Protracted pain and nursing care. *Nursing (UK)*, 1st series, *2*, 56.

JONES, J. (1982) Give and take, *Nursing Mirror, 154*:7, xiii.

LOCKSTONE, C. (1982) It's what the patient says it is. *Nursing Mirror, 154*:7, ii.

McCAFFERY, M. (1980) Understanding your patient's pain. *Nursing (US) 10*:9, 26.

MELLOR, D. & DIXON, K. (1982) Breaking free from pain. *Nursing Mirror, 154*:20, 49.

MEYER, T.M. (1982) Transcutaneous electrical nerve stimulation — relieving pain through electricity. *Nursing (US), 12*:9, 57.

MILES, J. (1980) Electrical stimulation. *Nursing Mirror, 150*:7, 46.

WEST, B.A. (1981) Understanding endorphins: our natural pain relief system. *Nursing (US) 11*:2, 50.

23 The therapeutic team

The focus, and key member, of the therapeutic team is the patient, and without his active participation in the overall treatment programme, the ultimate outcome will be marred. However intensive and united the care given by hospital nurses, doctors, physiotherapists, medical social workers, occupational therapists, speech therapists and dieticians and their community counterparts, it is the patient and his family who must continually cope with the residual problems that beset so many disorders of the nervous system.

THE NURSE

The nurse's role within neuromedicine and neurosurgery is complex and far reaching. She will be asked to deal with people of all ages and with different backgrounds: the newborn baby with hydrocephalus, the teenager with multiple injuries, a mother struck by multiple sclerosis, a breadwinner diagnosed as having a tumour and needing to undergo surgery, and the elderly person incapacitated by a cerebrovascular disorder.

The basic function of the nurse in caring for the head-injured patient is observation. More specifically, it is the patient's conscious level that must be closely monitored, particularly in the early stages when the patient is at his greatest danger of deterioration. Clear documentation of the nurse's findings and the use of a practical conscious level observation scale will determine any deterioration in the patient's condition.

Provision of physical bodily needs will be provided, especially in those patients with a compromised conscious level.

The nurse will accompany the patient during potentially hazardous and unpleasant investigative procedures, and will provide realistic reassurance and support. The patient preparing for major surgery will rely on the nurse for guidance and support. She must answer his questions honestly and sympathetically as far as her professional role will allow.

Observation following craniotomy and other surgical procedures is important. Deterioration may signify a collecting haematoma which will need to be dealt with quickly if the patient is to survive. Special needs following surgery will be attended to, e.g. a naso-gastric tube will be passed on those patients with a bulbar palsy, following posterior fossa surgery. Support for the family will be given by the nurse during what is a stressful and critical time for them.

The patient who is admitted to hospital with an unrelentless chronic neurological disorder will require a lot of physical and psychological support and advice. Some disorders follow a relapse/remission pattern and this can be very demoralising for the patient. Liaison with other members of the therapeutic team and community support on discharge, from NHS agencies and self-help groups, will be organised by the nurse. Patient and family teaching regarding medication compliance and altered life-style due to a disability will need to be performed, and the nurse is often the best person to do this.

It is required of the nurse to see that the patient's family is also supported during his illness. For some, hospitalisation of a bread-winner can be financially disastrous, and a talk with the medical social worker should be arranged. For others, it may mean long travelling distances and only getting to see the patient once a week, or not at all. When a child is hospitalised, it may be possible to arrange for the mother or father to stay as well.

The nurse also has a professional responsibility to keep abreast of new developments and maintain a high standard of teaching in the ward.

THE PHYSIOTHERAPIST

The physiotherapist will generally participate during most stages in the care of the neurological patient. More specifically, his or her function could be subdivided into three main areas:

   a.   passive treatment,
   b.   active treatment,
   c.   advisory.

Passive treatment

This is essentially work carried out by the therapist without active assistance from the patient. The most common form of this therapy is that of passive joint movement, which is carried out twice daily to the limbs of the comatosed or paralysed patient in order to help prevent joint and muscle contractures which would ultimately severely hamper continuing rehabilitation. Passive movements themselves are performed in two basic methods.

1. Anatomical movement:
   a. flexion and extension;
   b. abduction and adduction;
   c. internal and external rotation.
2. Patterns of movement: the entire limb is moved through a specific arc closely related to functional movement.

Positioning the limbs of the patient in bed is also very important, as this helps to reduce excessive muscle tone (very often extensor) and so aid in the prevention of contractures. The guidance of a physiotherapist can be invaluable when severe extensor posturing becomes an additional nursing problem. The position of the head can in many instances alter the posturing of both upper and lower limbs. Splints and other similar appliances have their value. However, some controversy does surround their use, and in many centres they are not used at all.

Chest care is a major part of the physiotherapist's function during the initial intensive care stage of patient management. The aims at this time are to ensure a clear airway, encourage adequate pulmonary function, and to stimulate a strong cough reflex. Various manipulations are performed on the patient to achieve this aim, but they are too numerous to explain in this text. Two further aspects of chest care need to be noted and the first is that of humidification. In a large number of cases, and especially those who have aspirated, humidification should always be incorporated with oxygen therapy and, if at all possible, the humidification should be nebulised for greater effect. The second, and equally important, point is that concerning the technique of 'bagging'. This is of undoubted value when a patient develops a lung or lobar collapse; however, it should not be undertaken in patients with raised intracranial pressure unless with great care and medical guidance.

Active treatment

This encompasses many forms of specific exercises, and in many instances follows methods laid down by various experts in the physiotherapy profession.

The major aim of the physiotherapist is to ensure that the patient regains or achieves the maximum level of functional independence. The initial examination and assessment of the patient provide the therapist with a base line from which continuing progress can be measured. From the early stages, a patient is asked to perform increasingly difficult levels of activity, the emphasis initially being geared towards sitting and rolling in order to achieve trunk control. Standing, even at an early stage, is an important activity as it stimulates the proximal muscles (i.e. hip/knee muscles) to stabilise the lower limb. Basically, movement is controlled from the body and out towards the limbs. A normal functioning hand would be useless unless we were able to stabilise and control the shoulder and elbow joints.

In order to achieve these motor or functional activities, the therapist makes use of many inherent postural and reflex mechanisms, at the same time stimulating many specific sensory modalities.

One of the initial forms of physiotherapy that is extremely useful in the early management of the neurological patient is that of hydrotherapy. The pool (which can vary in size) is maintained at a constant temperature of 35°C. In this warm and gravity-free environment, even the very weak and disabled patient can begin to re-educate muscle activity. During these early stages the patient is fitted with flotation aids, and is always assisted by the therapist.

Advice

Inevitably, some patients require a form of aid or appliance in order to gain their maximal level of independence. There are now many aids on the market, which can make the choice somewhat difficult. However, to overcome this difficulty, regular communication with the therapist can be of great value in the appropriate selection.

The physiotherapist should also be regularly available to offer and provide advice to the nursing staff on matters of posturing and movement, many of which are simple and ultimately result in less stress to the nurses and, most important of all, less discomfort to the patient during his rehabilitation period. Yet another important role of the physiotherapist is to offer advice and to counsel the relatives, many of whom are very distraught at the thought of a close relative being either physically or psychologically impaired. The relatives should, where possible, be taught to handle the patient physically and therefore to participate actively in his rehabilitation.

Finally, the rehabilitation of the neurological patient will run most effectively when all the professional groups involved have a true understanding of each others' role.

THE OCCUPATIONAL THERAPIST

Occupational therapy is treatment which includes the use of any activity, work or recreation, chosen specifically to aid recovery and resettlement and to help the patient with residual disability to live as full a life as possible. The main aims for patients suffering from neurological diseases are:

- *a.* to assess existing function;
- *b.* to improve physical and mental capacity;
- *c.* to help the patient cope with residual problems;
- *d.* to resettle the patient into the community.

Assessing existing function

In her initial assessment, the occupational therapist will use a variety of tests (for example, shape and colour recognition, body image and position in space, vision and hearing, hand and eye co-ordination) to establish if the patient has any perceptual difficulties. If so, details are conveyed to all the staff so that the situation is less stressful for the patient. Measurements of muscle strength, range of joint movements and sensory perception are carried out as appropriate.

Information regarding the patient's previous personality, educational achievements, work and social background is obtained from relatives or friends, and the home situation is carefully considered. Whether the patient's accommodation will be suitable for his future use is questioned, and an understanding of the relationships within the family is sought. The occupational therapist and the medical social worker liaise over this issue, which is often the determining factor as to whether resettlement is achieved smoothly or not at all.

Improving physical and mental capacity

Having assessed the patient, the occupational therapist plans a treatment programme with specific aims related to individual needs. These obviously vary tremendously, but the following are examples.

The severely physically impaired head injury patient

Provision for postural support, with, for example, a strategically padded wheelchair or geriatric chair, so that maximum function can be utilised is a vital, but often lengthy, task for the occupational therapist and physiotherapist. However, as a result, both speech and swallowing are facilitated, physiological systems are nearer the vertical, function of the upper limbs is encouraged (perhaps with the help of slings or ball-bearing supports), and the relatives see the patient as someone who might be about to do something rather than as an inanimate body lying in a bed. Aids can be provided to enable the patient to carry out several activities independently, e.g. turn over pages in a book, ring an alarm, and operate remote control equipment for television, radio and lights. The occupational therapist may also ensure that the patient receives maximum mental stimulation, e.g. by liaising with voluntary workers and arranging for delivery of daily newspapers.

The head injury patient with mainly mental problems

Treatment is carried out using carefully graded, simple tasks with which the patient will have been familiar in the past. Activities such as washing up, dressing, folding, copying and simple counting can help to improve concentration span, work and noise tolerance, and the ability to cope with spelling, vocabulary, arithmetic and money. The patient is gradually weaned from working in a quiet, relaxed atmosphere to undertaking a job in a noisy, busy workshop.

The patient with hemiplegia, multiple sclerosis or Parkinson's disease

Such patients benefit from tasks selected to improve muscular power, co-ordination, and range of movements in joints. Activities include remedial games such as draughts, noughts and crosses, and dominoes, in which grips and weights of the playing pieces are adapted to suit the patient. Bimanual occupations such as sanding, sawing and polishing can be assisted by slings and springs. The occupational therapist is also concerned with the construction of splints (wrist extensions, back slab, night-resting or lively) as needed. Patients with Parkinson's disease are helped by gross movements, e.g. using a bicycle or treadle fretsaw. A standing harness for balance practice enables the patient to carry out a task while improving his righting reflexes. Where function allows, constructive activities, e.g. stool seating and woodwork, are encouraged. Printing and weaving may be adapted by using pulley systems which arrange the work so that specific muscle groups are being exercised.

The patient's morale must be maintained and his achievements constantly emphasised. Not only does he require considerable help in coping with the activities of daily living, but he may need to be guided into new hobbies and interests before old pastimes become impossible. Multiple sclerosis patients are taught to conserve their energy and ensure safety in the home.

Helping the patient cope with residual problems

The occupational therapist must constantly evaluate the patient's capabilities and relate these to everyday needs. Independence must be encouraged and may involve the supply or design of aids, of which the following are some of the most commonly used.

Eating utensils. A plate guard, non-slip mat and cutlery with enlarged and/or angled handles are supplied as needed, and the nurse should make sure that the patient has his own aids for every meal.

Dressing equipment. Velcro fastenings, elastic laces and button hooks are useful, and dressing techniques should be reinforced daily by the nursing and auxiliary staff.

Bed aids. When power in one or both arms is good, the provision of a monkey pole or bed ladder enables the patient to haul himself into the sitting position. Raising the bed on blocks may allow the patient to get in and out of bed on his own.

Transfer devices. Transfer boards and mobile hoists are of great value for the severely disabled patient, particularly at bath time.

Bathroom and lavatory facilities. Bathing may be made easier and safer by the use of well-positioned handrails, a non-slip bath mat, or a stool in the bath. Likewise, the provision of wall rails and a raised seat in the lavatory encourages independence.

Writing implements. Felt-tip pens are easy to write with and can be given enlarged handles for patients with poor grip. Weighted sleeve cuffs may reduce tremor.

It is interesting and useful for the nurse to visit an occupational therapy department in order that the diversity of the equipment available to the disabled can be appreciated.

While a patient is being taught to use these aids, the opportunity arises for his relatives to become closely involved with rehabilitation. Through sorting out methods of coping with practical everyday activities, they can develop confidence in each other, which is an ideal foundation for the next stage of treatment.

Resettling the patient into the community

The occupational therapist is consulted as to whether the patient's abilities are sufficiently good to allow him to return to his previous home and work. Liaison with the community occupational therapist is established, and a home visit may be carried out so that the provision of adaptations, such as rails on the stairs and in the toilet areas, ramps and widened doorways, may be initiated and completed before the patient returns.

Treatment in specialised rehabilitation or industrial training and assessment centres is organised for some patients. The occupational therapists in these units work closely with the disablement resettlement officers.

THE SPEECH THERAPIST

The speech therapist is concerned with patients who are impaired in the ability to use an adequate system of communication. This may result from either the breakdown of an established process, for example damage following a cerebral vascular accident, or failure of a system to develop properly, such as language delay from hearing loss or mental retardation.

Language is a system of symbols that is used to understand and classify the environment and express feelings and experiences. It requires an intact memory because memories that cannot be expressed and language that cannot be remembered when needed are equally useless. Communication may be by speech, writing, reading or gesture as used by deaf people.

There are four basic groups of problems of communication.

1. Disturbances of voice (dysphonia) such as huskiness and loss of power.
2. Defects of rhythm, mainly stammering (stuttering).
3. Disorders of language (dysphasia) caused by a lesion in the part of the brain that deals with the understanding and use of language symbols.
4. Impairment of speech, such as poor articulation from cleft palate, muscle paresis (dysarthria) or hearing loss.

The last two groups are the most commonly encountered in diseases of the nervous system.

In the majority of people, whether they are left or right handed, the area that controls language is on the left cerebral hemisphere. Before the age of 5 years, the brain is still flexible and the right side may take over if the left is damaged, but after this a cerebral vascular accident, head injury or space-occupying lesion will disrupt the ability to manipulate and/or understand the language symbols, and long-term rehabilitation will be needed to ensure the maximum recovery. Skilled testing to elicit the fine difference of individual language damage must be undertaken so that the appropriate therapy is offered. Dysphasia may be comprehensive or expressive, as explained on page 14. Sometimes, dyspraxia is included in expressive dysfunction. Here, the patient can produce a word or action spontaneously but not voluntarily. However, when shown the first lip or tongue movement, this may act as a trigger and allow the patient subsequently to articulate the desired word or phrase.

Treatment of dysphasia, which consists of reteaching the patient the language he used before his illness, should be considered at an early stage. Each programme is carefully designed to assist the patient's specific difficulties, having first considered his language requirements and experience. A retired labourer and a middle-aged professional man are likely to have very different language backgrounds and future needs.

Although tape recorders, with or without a built-in visual system, may be used, the majority of the patients' therapy is with pen, paper and the speech therapist. Reading and writing are taught; the patient may need to learn to write with his left hand if he has a right hemiplegia. The patient is assessed for any visual and hearing defects so that these can be allowed for.

Therapy time varies; each session depends on the patient's tolerance, and the overall duration is governed by the extent of the permanent damage. A therapist may spend weeks with a severely dysphasic patient trying to improve simple understanding, e.g. picking out the correct object from two or three. A patient with a high-level loss affecting only the most complex and abstract language may need help that seems like sixth-form English lessons. Speech therapy often continues long after other treatments are complete, particularly in patients with strokes. Individual or group therapy is provided for out-patients and, where applicable and available, the therapists arrange attendance at a 'Stroke Club'.

Disorders of speech can be from misuse (usually psychological) or abnormality of the articulatory mechanism, i.e. lips, teeth, jaw, tongue, palate and facial muscles. The types of malfunctions encountered in neurological nursing are generally weakness of the speech musculature causing poor pronunciation and sometimes swallowing problems, depending on the site of the brain lesion. They can occur in conjuncture with language disturbances, e.g. right hemiparesis from a cerebral vascular accident or separately, as in motor neurone disease, Parkinson's disease or facial palsy. When therapy is indicated, the physiotherapist may endorse the work of the speech therapist. The first aim of treatment, which is based on muscle exercises and massage, is function and clarity, and the second is cosmetic. Mirrors are sometimes used to enable the patients to work alone. When appropriate, ice (cold acts as a stimulus) may be placed on the lips and external speech musculature to encourage movement. The swallowing muscles may be stimulated by stroking and brushing the neck under the chin.

Talking to a patient with communication problems requires not only care but skill, and a speech therapist should be consulted as to whether the patient is capable of attempting to say more than 'yes' or 'no'. Shouting or speaking as if the patient is simple or deaf must be avoided.

The inability to speak well can be, and usually is, humiliating and frustrating. The patient's communicative proficiency and self-confidence are both helped by constant encouragement, and a sensitive approach does much to promote adjustment to any residual impairment.

THE SOCIAL WORKER

The social worker's contribution to patient care is different from other roles in the hospital setting, in that it focuses on the social implications of illness rather than the medical aspects. The social worker learns of the patient's requirements from medical and nursing staff and keeps these in mind when looking at the patient and his family's social situation.

Many patients who have a chronic neurological condition face necessary changes to their life-style (loss of employment, change of status, e.g. breadwinner can no longer earn or housewife cannot manage usual household activities, enforced dependency). This has implications for the whole family, and the patient and his relatives need opportunities to discuss what these changes will mean in day-to-day terms and how to cope with the new situation. The social worker can give practical advice and assistance and at the same time help the family look at their emotional reactions to these enforced changes to their normal life. Anger, resentment, despair and frustration are commonly experienced by patient and family in such circumstances, and to learn that this is not unique to their family can in itself come as a great relief.

For the patient who sustains traumatic injury, the initial impact of the situation has most effect on the relatives. The social worker can offer help by assisting families to deal with their feelings of shock, fear and guilt, and help them cope with the practical matters which often arise at such times, such as the need for arranging care of children, care of an elderly person left alone, legal and financial affairs.

Patients tend now to have much more knowledge of what help and resources are available to them (welfare benefits, housing for the handicapped, day centres etc.) and may well initiate contact with a social worker themselves. Often, discussion of a practical matter affords the patient the opportunity to extend his enquiry to seeking advice on a more personal problem. Nurses perhaps have the closest contact with patients and can assist a diffident or anxious person to seek help where appropriate, by advising them of a social worker's presence and explaining how they might be helped. Being told that it is quite common to experience some problem or worry allied to illness, and that it is sensible to seek help, and not a demonstration of personal failure to cope, can, when done by a trusted nurse, greatly help unsure or inarticulate patients.

The social worker can contribute to patient care by indicating to nursing and medical colleagues the provisions and possibilities for social/community care which could be made available, in order that good planning for the patient's rehabilitation, care at home, or need for continuing institutional care can be carried out.

Neurological units with a regional catchment area can pose particular problems. Relatives who have had to leave their home area to be near a patient might require a social worker to help them find accommodation near to the hospital, or to help them make provision for care of other family members (or pets), and the maintenance of their household in their absence. When the patient is able to return to his home area, social workers can usefully enquire about any special local facilities, e.g. support groups, voluntary organisations, introduction to which could greatly benefit some patients and families. There are many local variations in the provision and delivery of both statutory and voluntary social services, and it is important that the patient and those concerned with his care are made aware of these. Often the needs of patients having a neurological or neurosurgical problem are not familiar to those in the community who will be trying to assist the patient and family at home. Staff from regional specialist units, including the social worker, can usefully contribute towards their patient's rehabilitation through discussion and liaison with colleagues in the community.

There is a place for social work in the intensive care setting where the patient's relatives can need much attention. This usually is left to the nursing staff, who very often have too many demands placed on them in giving direct care to the patient to have time to spend with relatives, who need maximum attention at the same time as the patient does, e.g. immediately after admission. The social worker can make time to spend with distressed relatives listening to them, dealing with some of their anxieties and demonstrating the therapeutic team's understanding of their needs, which can be a beginning towards the relieving of some of their distress.

THE DIETICIAN

Nutrition has a particular relevance to many neurological problems. The emphasis is on the team approach to patient care, and the dietician, with her specialist knowledge and expertise, has an important part to play. The main areas which involve the dietician arise with patients with physical feeding problems and those requiring nutritional support.

Physical feeding problems

Many neuromedical and neurosurgical patients have conditions which result in difficulty in chewing and/or swallowing. Examples of these are, myasthenia gravis, parkinsonism, bulbar palsy and patients with wired jaws following repair of facial fractures. These patients can easily become malnourished as a result of insufficient food intake. A simple modification of the consistency of food can help greatly to improve the patient's nutritional intake.

Soft diet. This is the first stage in the modification of ordinary food. The diet is essentially normal, but raw vegetables, fruit, or large chunks of meat are excluded as they require a lot of chewing.

Semi-solid diet. The foods used in this type of diet are similar in consistency to those given to a toddler. Meats are minced, fish flaked into a sauce, and egg dishes can also be used. Vegetables are usually mashed or puréed. The patient must have some degree of jaw movement to deal with these types of food, but hard chewing is not required.

Liquidised food. This is similar in consistency to weaning foods. Meats are liquidised with gravy, vegetables are puréed, and puddings should be smooth. These foods require some control of the mouth, but can be sucked and swallowed.

Fluids. An adequate intake of nutrients is difficult to achieve since this would involve the patient in consuming large volumes of fluid, so careful planning is necessary. Thin, strained soup, thin milk puddings, melted ice cream, milk, fortified milk drinks and fruit juices are all useful. Sometimes an energy and/or protein supplement will be added to the drinks to increase their nutritive value. A patient with wired jaws may only be able to cope with fluid foods.

It must be borne in mind that a patient requiring any of these dietary modifications must have adequate tongue movement and good lip closure. The speech therapist will be able to advise if necessary. Once a suitable diet is selected, it is important that the nurse continues to assess its suitability and, if necessary, modifies the diet as required.

Nutritional support

Any trauma to the body, whether by injury or surgery, results in a disturbance of the body's metabolism. As a result of better knowledge of the body's response to stress, and with the advances made in nutritional products, it is possible to cater for all the body's metabolic requirements.

It should be borne in mind that trauma results in an increased nutritional requirement and in these circumstances an adequate voluntary intake becomes difficult or indeed impossible to maintain. The consequences of not meeting the patient's requirements for energy and protein can be grave, since the body's reserves of these are limited and quickly depleted. If the situation is allowed to continue, it will result in a loss of total body weight, an increased susceptibility to infection, increased incidence of wound breakdown, hypoproteinaemic oedema and overall increased mortality.

Assessing the need for nutritional support

Data should be obtained in order to form an individual assessment of the patient's needs. If the patient has a visible weight loss or a poor food intake, he may be in need of some extra nutrition.

Appropriate measurements may include weight/height, mid-arm muscle circumference (MAMC), triceps skinfold thickness (TST), and serum albumin levels.

Recording the weight and height is one of the most reliable ways of assessing the patient, but unfortunately this is very difficult, for example in the case of the unconscious who cannot be weighed by traditional means. Mid-arm muscle circumference is obtained with a tape measure and can easily be performed on all patients. It gives an indication of the patient's protein reserves. The average measurement would be 23 cm in a male and 22 cm in a female.

Measurements of the triceps skinfold thickness (male = 10 mm, female = 13 mm) is made using skin calipers and provides an indication of the patient's fat stores.

A serum albumin less than 35 g/l may indicate poor protein status. These data are obtained at the onset to assess the need for nutritional support, and the tests are repeated at periodic intervals to ensure that the support is adequate.

Supplying the patient's nutrition

The patient's requirements for energy and protein can be supplied in a number of different ways: by oral supplementation, tube feeding or parenteral feeding. Where possible, the gastrointestinal tract, which is the natural route of entry for nutrients, should be used.

Oral supplementation. If it is considered possible for a patient to increase his oral intake voluntarily, then oral supplementation is used, e.g. fortified milk drinks, fruit juices with energy or protein supplements added, or proprietary sip feeds. The patient's intake should be carefully monitored to ensure that an increase is being achieved. If it falls below the desired amount, an alternative method of feeding must be considered.

Supplementary nasogastric feeding may be useful in this situation. The use of a fine-bore feeding tube will permit the patient to accept oral diet while the tube remains *in situ*.

Tube feeding. If supplementation of the diet becomes inadequate in the patient with a viable gastrointestinal tract, then total naso-gastric feeding should be initiated. This would then be the patient's only source of nutrition; therefore all the essential nutrients must be included in the feed in optimum amounts. The most important considerations for a tube feed are the fluid, protein and energy content.

The normal fluid requirement is 2–2.5 litres, and this may have to be increased if the patient is pyrexic. Some head-injured patients may be fluid restricted, and the volume of tube feed would have to be adjusted accordingly in consultation with the dietician: 1 g protein/kg of ideal body weight per day is required, and may be increased in the traumatised patient to 1.5 g protein/kg ideal body weight per day. Approximately 40 kilocalories/kg of ideal body weight per day are required. Variations occur which could mean some patients requiring between 2500 and 4000 kilocalories per day. The main sources of energy in a tube feed are fat and carbohydrate, the latter being the nutrient of choice since excessive fat may cause diarrhoea. The patient's requirements for electrolytes, vitamins, minerals and trace elements must also be included in the tube feed.

Method of administration. Where possible, continuous drip feeding should be the method of choice. The feed is contained in a reservoir, i.e. bag or bottle, and drips by gravity into the patient's feeding tube. This facilitates slow administration of the feed, giving the best chance of absorption and less likelihood of diarrhoea.

Pump-assisted feeding may be useful in the sensitive patient who requires finer control of delivery.

It may be necessary to feed a very restless patient by giving bolus feeds. A bolus feed may contain 100–400 ml of fluid and be given 3–4-hourly. This means that the feed is delivered at a much faster rate and may precipitate diarrhoea and vomiting.

Introduction of feed. Generally speaking, the volume and strength of a feed should be increased gradually over a few days. The following is an example of a suitable feeding regime.

Day 1	water	100 ml/hour	for 3 hours
	half-strength milk	100 ml/hour	for 3 hours
	full-strength milk	100 ml/hour	for 3 hours
	half-strength feed	100 ml/hour	for 15 hours
Day 2	full-strength feed	100 ml/hour	for 24 hours
Day 3	full-strength feed	125 ml/hour	for 24 hours

If at any stage the patient does not tolerate the feed, one should return to a previous stage in the feeding regime. There are several reasons why a patient may develop diarrhoea while being tube fed.

1. Feed opened or made up for more than 24 hours.

2. Amount of fluid given per feed is too much for the patient.
3. Feed may have been given when too cold. It is recommended to give feed which is at room temperature.
4. The feed may be too concentrated, resulting in osmotic diarrhoea.
5. The patient may have a 'sterile gut' due to high doses of antibiotics. In this case, natural unsweetened yogurt given as a nasogastric feed may help recolonise the gut.
6. Chest physiotherapy is being administered too soon following the feed.

If all these points have been checked and diarrhoea still persists, it is best controlled with a suitable drug, e.g. diphenoxylate hydrochloride (Lomotil).

Content of tube feed. There is a large variety of nutritionally complete, commercially prepared feeds available, and these are being used increasingly in many hospitals. The advantages of these are that they are complete, ready to use, sterile, of low osmolarity, pass easily down a fine-bore tube, and can be adapted to suit individual requirements.

An alternative to commercial products is a made-up feed, which may be used in some hospitals. This can be a mixture of several products but may require additional vitamins and minerals during preparation. These feeds may be of higher osmolarity, but should be perfectly acceptable if administered slowly. It should be noted that there is a greater risk of contamination during the preparation of these feeds.

The use of liquidised meals for tube feeding is no longer considered desirable. In order to liquidise the meal into a suitable consistency, vast quantities of fluid would have to be used which the patient would not tolerate.

Parenteral feeding. If nasogastric feeding becomes contraindicated, e.g. due to persistent returns of large volumes of gastric aspirate, then parenteral feeding is indicated. The nutritional considerations for parenteral feeding are the same as those for enteral feeding. An intravenous meal of nitrogen, energy, water, electrolytes and vitamins has to be provided which has to suit the patient's individual nutritional requirements.

Appendix

The criteria used in the United Kingdom to determine cerebral death are those laid down by the Conference of Medical Royal Colleges and their Faculties of the United Kingdom. Before tests can be performed to establish cerebral death, certain pre-conditions must be fulfilled.

These pre-conditions are that the patient must be in deep coma and apnoeic (supported by artificial ventilation), that there must be definitive knowledge of the irremediable structural brain damage leading to this catastrophe, and that there are no reversible causes of brainstem depression present; such causes include the administration of depressant or neuromuscular blocking drugs and the presence of hypothermia or metabolic disturbances.

Testing for cerebral death involves determining the presence or absence of reflex responses. This entails checking the pupillary reactions to light, the corneal and gag reflexes, and the cranial nerve motor responses to deep painful stimuli. Eye movement is checked for after irrigating the ear with ice-cold water, ascertaining first that the ear drum can be visualised. A positive reaction will consist of movement of the eye to the side that was stimulated; this implies that the oculovestibular reflex is intact and that the brainstem is still functioning. Absence of eye movement implies that the brainstem is not functioning. The patient is disconnected from the ventilator for a period of time, with oxygenation maintained, long enough to allow the $PaCO_2$ to rise to a threshold level. In many centres 50 mmHg or above is an acceptable level in a normocapnic patient.

If the patient fulfils these criteria he is considered brain dead. However, before supportive measures are withdrawn, a second, clinically independent, doctor will review the patient and repeat the criteria. The time interval between testing can be as short as 30 minutes or as long as 24 hours. If the patient again fulfils the criteria on the second occasion then, when the appropriate forms are signed and dated, this is, in medico-legal terms, the time of death.

The performance of these tests for brain death on patients who have no chance of recovery allows death to occur with dignity and avoids prolonging the agony for relatives. The effects, both long and short term, upon nursing staff who care for these patients are as yet unresearched but are almost certainly demoralising and upsetting. These criteria also permit the release of essential equipment for use by other patients with potentially retrievable conditions, or who may be denied access to the unit because of a shortage of beds.

Mention should be made of organ transplantation. The tests for brain death are *not* performed for the sake of obtaining organs for donations; however, in a few select cases, organ transplantation may be considered and this will be discussed with the relatives at the appropriate moment.

FURTHER READING

JENNET, W.B. (1983) Brain death. *The Practitioner, 227*:1377, 451.
JENNET, W.B. (1976) Diagnosis of brain death. *Lancet, ii*, 1069.

Index

Myositis, 231, 236–237
related nursing skills, 237
Myotonia, 235

Nails, care of, 97
Nasogastric tube, feeding, 86, 95, 114,
128–129, 173, 200, 241
Nerve(s)
conduction time, 54, 242
cranial, see Cranial nerves
roots, 49, 283
synapse, see Synapse
Neuralgia
glossopharyngeal, 253
post-herpetic, 252–253
trigeminal, 250–252, 281
related nursing skills, 251–252
Neural tube, 269
Neurofibroma, neurinoma,
neurilemmoma, see Neuroma
Neuroleptanalgesia, 41
Neurological examination, 12–27
assessment of intellectual function,
13–15
equipment, 26–27
specific questions, 12–13
Neurological observations, 5–12, 39,
41, 85
in coma, 94
in hydrocephalus, 278
indications for, 31, 80, 170, 189
Neuroma, 26
acoustic, 134–135, 140–141
Neuropathy, 239, 258–259
causes, 239, 258–259
effects, 24, 229
investigations, 54, 259
Neurosyphilis, 124, 266
treatment, 125
Neurotransmitter, 214
Non-accidental injury, 85
Nuclear magnetic resonance, 3, 56
Nucleus pulposus, 149
Nurse, role of, 287–288
activities of daily living, 2, 4–5, 186
assessment, 2, 100
care plans, 2, 4, 100, 221
evaluation, 2, 100
history, 2
implementation, 2, 100
Nursing Process, 2–3
Nystagmus, 18, 256
in cerebellar disturbance, 204, 230

Occipital lobe, 182, 193
Occlusion of cerebral arteries, 124, 185
Occupational therapist, 183, 213, 228,
248, 291–297
Oculomotor nerve, see Cranial nerves
Oedema, cerebral, 70, 133, 171, 175,
182
Olfactory nerve, see Cranial nerves
Oligoclonal bands, 205
Ophthalmoscopy, 17
Opisthotonus, 112
Optic chiasma, compression, 136
Osteomyelitis, 163, 176

Paget's disease, 29
Pain, 281
back, see Backache
control of, 98
head, see Headache
limb(s), 122, 126, 155, 253, 283
muscle, 122, 128, 236
neck, 149
perception disturbances, 125, 253,
254
procedures for relief, 251, 253,
282–284
referred, 149
Painful stimuli, 8, 9, 10, 12
Palliative treatment, 74, 282–284
related nursing skills in pain relief,
284–285
Palsies
carpal tunnel, 260
common peroneal nerve, 261
femoral nerve, 261
plantar nerve, 261
post-tibial nerve, 261
pressure, 259–261
radial nerve, 260
sciatic nerve, 261
ulnar nerve, 260
Papilloedema, 45, 61, 274
Paraesthesiae, 250, 257
Paralysis, 218
flaccid, 22, 122, 126, 159, 219
periodic, 238
related nursing skills, 127–129,
221–229
spastic, 22, 220
spina bifida, 269–272
Paraplegia (paresis)
causes, 116, 124, 145, 163, 219
clinical features, 220